Health, Human Rights and Ethics

Health, Human Rights and Ethics

A Sociological Study in Hospital Setting

Ramesh Kumar Sangwan

RAWAT PUBLICATIONS
Jaipur • New Delhi • Bangalore • Guwahati • Kolkata

ISBN 978-81-316-0911-8

The publication of this book was financially supported by the ICSSR. The responsibility for the facts stated, opinions expressed, or conclusions reached, is entirely that of the author and that the ICSSR accepts no responsibility for them.

ICSSR Consultant: Professor Poornima Jain, Dayalbagh University, Department of Sociology, Dayalbagh, Agra.

Published by
Prem Rawat for **Rawat Publications**
Satyam Apts, Sector 3, Jawahar Nagar, Jaipur 302 004 (India)
Phone: 0141 265 1748 / 7006 Fax: 0141 265 1748
E-mail: info@rawatbooks.com
Website: www.rawatbooks.com

New Delhi Office
4858/24, Ansari Road, Daryaganj, New Delhi 110 002
Phone: 011 2326 3290

Also at *Bangalore, Guwahati* and *Kolkata*

Typeset by Rawat Computers, Jaipur
Printed at Nice Printing Press, New Delhi

To My Teacher
Professor Madhu Nagla

Contents

Abbreviations

AIIMS	All India Institute of Medical Sciences
AMC	Academic Medical Centres
ANC	Antenatal Care
BAMS	Bachelor of Ayurvedic Medicine and Surgery
BDS	Bachelor of Dental Surgery
CHC	Community Health Centre
DG	Director General
DOTS	Directly Observed Treatment Short Course
EMRI	Emergency Management and Research Institute
EMS	Emergency Medical Services
FMRAI	Federation of Medical Representative Association of India
JSA	Jan Swasthya Abhiyan
GDP	Gross Domestic Production
GoI	Government of India
HCMA	Haryana Civil Medical Services Association
HCS	Health Care System
HLEG	High Level Expert Group
HRM	Human Resource Management
MBBS	Bachelor of Medicine, Bachelor of Surgery
MD	Doctor of Medicine

MDG	Millennium Development Goals
MLC	Medico Legal Case
MRP	Maximum Retail Price
NCAER	National Council of Applied Economic Research
NFHS	National Family Health Survey
NHP	National Health Policy
NSSO	National Sample Survey Organization
OPD	Out Patient Department
PHC	Primary Health Centre
PPP	Public Private Partnership
RCHP	Reproductive and Child Health Programme
SAE	Serious Adverse Events
SC	Sub Centre
TNMSC	Tamil Nadu Medical Services Corporation
TOI	*Times of India*
UHC	Universal Health Coverage
UNICEF	United Nations Children's Fund
VHAI	Voluntary Health Association of India
WDR	*World Development Report*
WHR	*World Health Report*
WHO	World Health Organization

Preface

The research process was an important learning experience not only in terms of techniques of fieldwork and concepts in operation but also in terms of human relations. It was difficult to get exact details from patients and doctors about the institution or medical practices but we managed to convince them that this might affect free communication and got permission to meet inpatients on our own.

This is only one side of the story. On many occasions we also received a lot of support from some doctors and patients who had shown interest and enthusiasm in our research, even though they were not aware of the details of my research. Some of the doctors and the patients even did not mind to openly give their critical views on medical system and the condition of the hospital.

This human relation brings me to express my heartfelt gratitude to several people who actively supported me throughout this research. When I look back, I realize that without the support of my teachers, family members and friends, this work would not have been possible.

First of all, I would like to thank my esteemed supervisor, Prof. Madhu Nagla, Head, Department of Sociology, Maharshi Dayanand University, Rohtak, who has constantly guided and supported me. I have learnt a lot while working with her. Her erudite knowledge, insightful comments and fruitful suggestions helped me to finish this thesis. I especially thank her for giving me sufficient time and lending me unconditional support whenever I needed. She also helped me in understanding the issues and conceptualizing theories. In times of difficulty, my supervisor was always just a call away, generously inviting me home and sharing her expert advice. I enjoyed her excellent professional visibility and enormous affection which made me fearless and confident whenever I consulted her. I am highly fortunate and privileged to have worked under her supervision.

I express my sincere gratitude to all the faculty members of Department of Sociology M.D. University, Rohtak including Prof. Kanwar Chauhan, Prof. Jitender Prasad, Prof. Des Raj, Prof. Supriti and Dr Neerja Ahlawat for their kind suggestions and cooperation.

I am thankful to Madam Darshna and Mr Dharemender, Department of Sociology and Dr Satish Malik, Librarian, M.D. University, Rohtak for providing journals, internet and other facilities.

I express my best regards to doctors, patients and paramedical staffs members, who helped me during my fieldwork and provided me all possible data and information.

I must convey my special gratitude and appreciation to my family members and parents. Naresh Kumar and Dinesh Kumar (Manager, Punjab National Bank) despite being my younger brothers they played the role of elder brothers and supported me in all possible ways with their keen sense of understanding me and unhesitatingly providing me all help and encouragement to complete this work. My wife, Sumanlata, has assisted me a lot. I am highly obliged to her. I express my gratitude to my daughter Muskan and my son Nitin who supported me considerably during the course of my study; they deserve my best blessings. I would also thank Prof. B.K. Nagla and Sh. Pradeep Kasni (IAS) for their valuable suggestions in my research.

I am extremely thankful to my colleagues who supported me in my research work. I also express my sincere gratitude to my friends Ankit Singh Bhyan, Dr Ravinder Kumar Sheoran, Dr Vipin Sangwan, Dr Kapil Sangwan, Dr Manjeet Singh, Maj. Vivek Sangwan, Kuldeep Singh Panghal, Rajesh Phogat, and Mrs Pankaj. Last but not the least, thanks to my friend Capt. Ajeet Sangwan, his love and smile have give me special strength. Without naming each of them individually, I wish to acknowledge my grateful thanks to all my friends.

Lastly, I would like to thank God for everything.

Ramesh Kumar Sangwan

1

Introduction

> The world needs a global health guardian, a custodian of values, a protector and defender of health, including the right to health.
>
> —Dr Margaret Chan, Director-General, WHO

Health and well-being are deeply personal matters. Nothing is more intimate than the experience of conceiving and bearing a child, and giving birth to a unique human being; none of us can share another's fear or pain; and death itself is something we cannot share, however real the grief we suffer. The right to health means that governments must generate conditions in which everyone can be as healthy as possible. Such conditions range from ensuring availability of health services, healthy and safe working conditions, adequate housing and nutritious food. The right to health does not mean the right to be healthy.

The right to health care is primarily a claim to an entitlement, a positive right, not a protective fence. As entitlement rights are contrasted with privileges, group ideals, societal obligations, or acts of charity, and once legislated they become claims justified by the laws of the state (Chapman, 1993). The emphasis thus needs to shift from 'respect' and 'protect' to focus more on 'fulfil'. For the right to be effective, optimal resources that are needed to fulfil the core obligations have to be made available and utilized effectively.

I

Right to Health

The concept of right to health as a human right has recently emerged as a result of ever-growing consciousness about the dignity of human life, all over the world. Health care is considered as a socio-medical concept which implies that whatever is medically possible to promote the physical and mental well-being of the patient must be done. Right to health and health care is a fundamental right under Article-21 of the Constitution of India. This has also been emphasized by the Supreme Court of India in many of its rulings.

In *State of Haryana vs. Smt Santara* in a judgement delivered in 2000, the Supreme Court upheld the judgement of the High Court awarding compensation to Mrs Santara, who gave birth to a daughter in spite of a sterilization operation carried on her earlier. This is one of the cases of negligence during the sterilization operations. A poor labourer woman, who already had many children and had opted for sterilization, became pregnant and gave birth to a female child in spite of the sterilization operation that obviously, had failed. Smt Santra, the victim of the medical negligence, filed a suit for recovery of ₹ 2 lakh as damages for medical negligence, which was decreed for a sum of ₹ 54,000 with interest at the rate of 12 per cent per annum from the date of institution of the suit till the payment of the decretal amount (Hiremath and Mahabal, 2007).

This Article of the Constitution casts a special obligation on the state to protect citizen's life from medical and other forms of negligence. The Constitution guarantees fundamental rights to its people. Article 21 gives the citizens the Right to Life. As with all fundamental rights, the Right to Life is justiciable. Many other obligations, required to produce an egalitarian society, are enshrined in the Constitution and are listed under Directive Principles of State Policy. These include Article 47, 39 and 38, which argue for the need to raise the level of nutrition, enhance standards of living and improve public health. They also make a case for social justice and sustainable livelihoods. The right to health has been defined as the 'right to the enjoyment of a variety of facilities, goods, services and conditions necessary for the realization of the highest attainable standard of health' (CESCR, 2000).

History of Health Rights

Historically speaking, the right to health has roots in the 19th century public health movement in Europe and the US which produced sanitation reforms designed to reduce the burden of infectious disease. These reform efforts helped to solidify the belief that governments had a fundamental duty to provide for and protect the public health. In the Human Rights revolution, the government's duty in the health fields was translated into the right to health (Fidler, 1999).

Various meanings are attached to a right. Right is the permission to do something that is secured and protected by law. Still other definitions associate a right with conditional duty that binds only on the condition that the beneficiary chooses to have it exercised. There is something to recommend in each of these interpretations of the meaning of right to health care. Patients have right to be informed about the benefits and risks of medical procedure, but they are not required to exercise the right. Right is protected by society or secured by law to the individual (Barry, 1982).

Today in the era of globalization where public services are slowly being privately operated and open to market forces, access to them becomes a correlate of income distribution in which the poorer sectors have to fend for themselves in an increasingly unequal society.

India's legal framework is dualist (as against monist). International laws related to rights cannot be transformed and applied in the country unless there is appropriate domestic legislation. In 2000 with the launch of the *Jan Swasthya Abhiyan* (JSA) People's Health Initiative in India, civil society groups sought to prioritize the right to health and health care on its agenda. During the campaign for the right to health care, it was realized that in order to effectively use the various relevant judgements to realize the right to health as a fundamental right, there was a need to create supportive legal documentation.

The Indian Constitution provides a framework for a welfare/socialist pattern of development. While civil and political rights are enshrined as Fundamental Rights that are justiciable, social and economic rights like health, education, livelihoods, etc. are provided in the Directive Principles for the State and hence not justiciable. The latter comes under the domain of planned development, which the State steers through the Five-Year Plans and other development policy initiatives.

The right to health in all its forms and at all levels contains the following interrelated and essential elements:

(a) *Availability*: Functioning public health and health care facilities, goods and services, as well as programmes, have to be available in sufficient quantity within the State party. The precise nature of the facilities, goods and services will vary depending on numerous factors, including the state party's developmental level. They will include, however, the underlying determinants of health, such as safe and potable drinking water, adequate sanitation facilities, hospitals, clinics and other health-related buildings, trained medical and professional personnel receiving domestically competitive salaries and essential drugs, as defined by the WHO Action Programme on Essential Drugs.

(b) *Accessibility*: Health facilities, goods and services have to be accessible to everyone without discrimination, within the jurisdiction of the State party. Accessibility has four overlapping dimensions:

   (i) *Non-discrimination*: Health facilities, goods and services must be accessible to all, especially the most vulnerable or marginalized sections of the population, in law and in fact, without discrimination on any of the prohibited grounds.

   (ii) *Physical accessibility*: Health facilities, goods and services must be within safe physical reach for all sections of the population, especially vulnerable or marginalized groups, such as ethnic minorities and indigenous populations, women, children, adolescents, older persons, persons with disabilities and persons with HIV/AIDS. Accessibility also implies that medical services and underlying determinants of health, such as safe and potable water and adequate sanitation facilities, are within safe physical reach, including in rural areas. Accessibility further includes adequate access to buildings for persons with disabilities.

   (iii) *Economic accessibility (affordability)*: Health facilities, goods and services must be affordable for all. Payment for health care services, as well as services related to the underlying determinants of health, has to be based on the principle of equity, ensuring that these services, whether privately or publicly provided, are affordable for all, including socially disadvantaged groups. Equity demands that poorer households should not be disproportionately burdened with health expenses as compared to richer households.

(iv) *Information accessibility*: Accessibility includes the right to seek, receive and impart information and ideas concerning health issues. However, accessibility of information should not impair the right to have personal health data treated with confidentiality.

(c) *Acceptability*: All health facilities, goods and services must be respectful of medical ethics and culturally appropriate, i.e. respectful of the culture of individuals, minorities, peoples and communities, sensitive to gender and life-cycle requirements, as well as being designed to respect confidentiality and improve the health status of those concerned.

(d) *Quality:* Along with being culturally acceptable, health facilities, goods and services must also be scientifically and medically appropriate and of good quality. This requires, inter alia, skilled medical personnel, scientifically approved and unexpired drugs and hospital equipment, safe and potable water, and adequate sanitation (CESCR, 2000).

The right to health requires doing more than merely providing for comprehensive systems of health care delivery and insurance. It obligates them to undertake measures aimed at promoting individual and community health and at preventing diseases, to remove other external causes of morbidity and mortality, to eliminate health inequalities and to improve the conditions that may hamper achievement of the highest attainable level of health. The right to health is interdependent with many other human rights. The human right to health includes:

- The human right to the highest attainable standard of physical and mental health, including reproductive and sexual health.
- The human right to equal access to adequate health care and health related services, regardless of sex, race or other status.
- The human right to equitable distribution of food.
- The human right to an adequate standard of living and adequate housing.
- The human right to access to safe drinking water and sanitation.
- The human right to a safe and healthy environment.

- The human right to a safe and healthy workplace and to adequate protection for pregnant women in work that is proven to be harmful to them.
- The human right to education and access to information relating to health, including reproductive health and family planning to enable couples and individuals to decide freely and responsibly all matters of reproduction and sexuality.
- The human right of the child to an environment appropriate for physical and mental development (www.pdhre.org).

Government hospitals, health centres and dispensaries where services are free or rendered on payment of charges would also fall within the ambit of the law and the recipient of free services also becomes consumer, the apex court has ruled. The same interpretation is extended to private hospitals and clinics too. In fact, while making a case for treating patients who receive free service taken at par with those who pay for the service at government as well as private hospitals (*The Times of India*, 1995). Following case gives an idea about the equal law for private and government medical care facility.

A slum dweller from Parmat area, Alka, who had appealed to the court that the government either bear her medical expenses or she be allowed euthanasia, was shifted from Lucknow's Sanjay Gandhi Post Graduate Institute of Medical Sciences to AIIMS on 5 October. 'After keeping her under observation and carrying out regular check-ups for 21 days, including her mental health, the doctors at AIIMS said that they did not have facilities for her treatment and that she should be taken to private hospital – Christian Medical College, Vellore – where the treatment would take approximately ₹ 20 lakh', said Alka's brother Brajesh Tiwari. Her treatment includes a bone marrow transplant. The officials also told Brajesh that the government cannot intervene with the treatment at a private hospital (*The Hindu*, 2011A).

The principal objective of the medical profession is to render service to humanity with full respect for the dignity of profession and man. Physicians should merit the confidence of patients entrusted to their care, rendering to each a full measure of service and devotion. Physicians should try continuously to improve medical knowledge and skills and should make available to their patients and colleagues the benefits of their professional attainments. The physician should practise methods of healing founded on scientific basis and should not associate professionally with anyone who violates this principle. The honoured ideals of the medical profession imply that the responsibilities of the physician extend not only to individuals but also to society (Medical Council of India, 2002).

The debate *'Right to Health'* surrounding the implementation of the Human Right to health is fresh and full of possibilities for the developing world. In fact, India has been able to create a legal mechanism whereby the right to health can be protected and enforced. The early 1997s witnessed a watershed in Human Right litigation with the *Keshavanand Bharti v. State of Kerala* ushering in an unprecedented period of progressive jurisprudence following the reorganization by the court that Directive Principles for State Policy should enjoy the same status as 'traditional' fundamental rights. At the same time standing rules were relaxed in order to promote public interest litigation and access to justice. So there were two developments in 1980s, which led to increase in health related litigations (Khan, 1995).

Private provision of health care is an important constituent of the health care delivery system in India and its role has increased considerably over time. Studies show that health care services provided by this sector are used not just by the affluent classes; a large number of poor people use them and have exhibited their preferences in approaching private doctors for their health problems. The growth of the private sector raises a number of concerns most of which stem from reasons of market failure. The State is supposed to play an important role in regulating this sector but it has so far remained passive (Bhat, 1993).

II

Right to Health Care: Some Approaches

Article 12 of the International Covenant on Economic, Social and Cultural Rights (1966) recognized that 'the right of every citizen is one of the highest attainable standards of physical and mental health'. While activists, non-governmental organizations, and scholars have made significant progress in promoting a human rights approach to the health and the field of health and human rights more generally (Mann et al., 1994). The question of a philosophical and conceptual foundation – a theory for the right to health through the cracks that emerge from an interdisciplinary intersection of medical ethics, international relations, international human rights law, health policy, health law and public health law.

The most important becoming on the right to health is medical ethics. 'Right to health care' implies on its face, a right to certain services; by contrast, 'a right to health' seems to imply a right to be healthy, which is an impossible standard (Hessler and Buchanan, 2002).

There are certain human right approaches, which help us to understand the importance of health care in the society. Below we will discuss them:

(i) *Utilitarianism and Health Policy:* Under utilitarianism, a right to health care would be justified if contributed to the overall maximum of net social utility. It would also be changeable if utility is changed. The types of health care services allocated would be those that maximized net social utility. Utilitarianism takes the principle of utility as absolute and does not necessarily give health a special place in that theory. In addition, utilitarianism accounts for aggregate welfare without taking note of the distributional concerns over benefits and burdens in society. There are no moral limits on measures to increase utility. Utilitarianism tolerates large inequalities to increase total or average net social utility. Utilitarianism also omits freedom as a good in itself and concentrates on achievements alone; it ignores value not reflected in measured utility. However, utility does not give us a good picture related to well-being in functional terms. This makes interpersonal comparison of utility difficult in health policy (Ruger, 2013).

(ii) *Communitarian Approach:* Communitarian approach of justice, as put forth by Sandel (1982) and Walzer (1990), offer a relative account of justice and health care and public health whereby the provision of health care is justified by the shared expression of values in a given community. There is no single principle of justice that governs the distribution of all social goods. Instead, under this theory, societies construct principles internally by the people as they evolve politically and constitute distinct 'spheres of justice' (Walzer, 1990).

(iii) *The Libertarian Perspective:* Libertarian theories of justice, as advocated by Robert Nozick (1974) would deny altogether any societal obligation to provide medical care or health insurance on other health determinants to all because the increased taxes required would infringe on individual liberties. Libertarianism takes the principle of liberty as absolute and does not give to health any special standing. Libertarian perspective supports national laws that guarantee negative freedoms, but in general opposes the redistribution of resources required to fulfil positive rights.

(iv) *Egalitarian Rights-based Theory:* It has been put forward by Daniels and Sabin (2002) who argue for a right to health care on the basis of 'equality of opportunity'. It proposes that social institutions affecting health care distribution should be arranged, as far as possible, to allow each person to achieve a fair share of the normal range of opportunities present in that society. The normal range of opportunity is determined by the range of life plans that a person could reasonably hope to pursue, given his or her talents or skills (Beauchamp and Childress, 2001). Under this theory, the social obligation to provide health care is different and prior to the social obligation to provide other primary goals. Although Daniels claims priority for health care and insulates it from other social goods, this theory does not discriminate among the different types of health care that society is obliged to provide its citizen under an 'equality of opportunity approach'. It is easy to see how this approach can be problematic given the widespread and seemingly limitless array of factors that limit opportunity.

(v) *Capability Approach:* Ruger (2013) points out that egalitarian right-based approach would increase the supply or access to health care but not necessarily achieve social justice. Thus, Ruger offers an account of capability and takes health as a focal object of justice and efficiency in health policy and human rights. Health capabilities should be the central focal variable for assessing the equality and efficiency of health policy and law. More specifically, universal attention to people's capability to avert premature mentality and address avoidable morbidity should be the morally centred or prior objective of health policy and law. This moral and social obligation is universal – applying to all human lives, irrespective of class, gender, race, ethnicity, sexual orientation, or community. The focus on central health capabilities – the capability to avoid premature mortality and address escapable critically important functioning up to certain minimally adequate levels. As Sen (2004) notes, there is a 'particular moral and political importance' that is associated with fulfilling these well-recognized and urgent claims. According to capability approach, whether a group or person is a 'worse-off' or 'well-off' cannot be determined by access to health care or other primary goods. The information does not 'go deep enough in imaging the impediments to functioning that are actually prevalent in many human lives (Nussbaum, 1997). Thus, capability approach looks into people's capability to flourish as an end of political activity and provides an analytical framework to address questions of justice and efficiency in public policy in a way that other approaches do not.

The emphasis on heterogeneity of patient's for right to health because it provides a rationale for treating individuals differently. For example, children require different resources than adults to achieve optional physical and mental functioning. Thus, a newborn with phenomena may require hospitalization, antibiotics and defensive monitoring, whereas an adult would likely regain full pulmonary function with no hospitalization and low dosages of antibiotics. Similarly, a person with disability would require more resources than one without a disability to achieve the same capability to function, in the same way a man in a wheelchair needs an appropriately designed ramp to get into his workplace. Consider also the nutritional requirements of children, who need different types of calories than adults because they are growing, and pregnant women, who must take in adequate quantities of certain vitamins (e.g. folic acid) and nutrients to ensure normal foetal development. As Dreze and Sen (1989) show, the relationship between food intake and nutritional adequacy varies greatly with metabolic rate, body size, gender, pregnancy, age, climate, epidemiological characteristics and other factors.

On the account of capability and health, using preferences or utilities to evaluate health interventions will not necessarily produce allocations that serve the array of health functioning, health needs and health capabilities in a given society. Health preferences might be weak or health utilities might be low for certain objectively important health functioning, for example, in some cultures, devolution of women might diminish preferences for maternal health during and after pregnancy. In these cases, allocations will differ from those based on health capabilities, which invoke health functioning and health needs as objectively important criteria for resource allocation. So, on this view, safe motherhood in all countries is valued as an essential human functioning. Functioning, as opposed to utilities or preferences, also may lend themselves better to interpersonal comparison. And, as Sen notes, many types of functioning can be seen distinctly from their assessment (Sen, 1993).

The capability approach also has component of opportunity and process. The opportunity aspect judges public policy in terms of its impact on individual's substantive freedoms or capabilities to choose a life they have reason to value. Thus, public policy must be concerned with the opportunities individuals have to achieve valued outcomes. Applying this to health, health policies would be evaluated by their impact on individual's health capabilities and health functioning, selected and stated according to generally accepted standards. Developing institutions to maintain and improve health should reflect the influence of the public participating in social choice and decision-making.

Thus, capability approach focuses primarily on 'the individual as a member of the public' and as a participant in economic, social and political actions (Sen, 1993). Applying this principle to health, one would need to account for information asymmetry and the fact that individual might need assistance from experts. In this case, as with Aristotelian view, there would also be a role for physicians to share decision-making with patients. Enabling patients to make their own decisions as agents of their own health, however, is essential (Ruger, 2006).

From an ethical point of view, as Sen notes, the obligation of individuals and by extension of duty of states – requires them to address threats to individual's human rights (Sen, 1988). Sen applies Immanuel Kant's category of duties known as 'imperfect obligations' to human rights analysis as the basis for this obligation. Determining the extent and scope of such claims – for example, in applying this viewpoint to health – our perfect and imperfect obligations to respect, protect, and fulfil individual's right to health requires a framework of normative reasoning. Such reasoning involves dialogue about the ethical dimensions of health and health policy and the need for collective action through public financing, regulation, and in some cases, provision of services (Ruger, 2013).

III

Medical Ethics

The obligations of individuals to respect, protect and fulfil individual's right to health require a framework of narrative reasoning. This reasoning involves dialogue about the ethical dimensions of health. Most of our personal and professional attitudes stem from handful of values. There are four main sources from which we derive our values: experience, culture, science and religion. Our values are shaped by experience. Those who have felt the sting of discrimination may become champions of fair and just treatment. Health professionals who have been patients themselves can become highly sensitized to patient's rights. The values we hold as individuals and as groups are inseparable from the continuous changing experiences of our lives. Much of our experience is vicarious, we learn by watching and listening to other people. What others have experienced or are experiencing are powerful influences in ordering our personal values.

Each of us has a value system that is unique. Nonetheless, our individual values originate from the core value of our culture. Our culture offers variety of positions on these issues that can affect ones practice as a clinician. For example, ignoring a person's feelings of privacy or being insensitive to his or her religious beliefs, not being considerate of a person's reservation about confidentiality and informed consent, or disagreeing about how much of a person's welfare check should be allocated to health care, can affect the type of relationship that can be established between a client and helper (Coleman, 1974).

The practice of medicine has a special characteristic not found in so pronounced manner in other occupations. Doctors deal directly, and at the time when a person is most vulnerable, with the immediate issues of life and death, health and illness. The patient is heavily dependent upon the technical knowledge and integrity of the doctor. The doctor thus has a unique involvement with the patient, but this relationship, between doctor and patient, is not balanced. The patient's attitude is a complex of trust (which comes from perceived competence and integrity of doctor) and, paradoxically, also that of distrust which comes from the state of uncertainty and vulnerability (Jesani, 1995).

The feelings and expression of sympathy is an integral part of the approach to a patient. But sympathy has its pitfalls. The mere expression of sympathy, however genuine and heartfelt, is far from being therapeutic. Sympathy is an emotional response to be used under conscious intellectual control. It may act as a barrier to effective communication between doctor and patient, and secondly, it may be used by the patient for his own ends: the doctor may be manoeuvred into actions which may serve only to foster the patient's neurosis and be the reverse of therapeutic (Goel and Kumar, 1990).

Health promotion initiatives and in particular health education programmes, have two major ethical concerns: liberty and justice. With regard to liberty, they assert that health promotion programmes should be carefully examined with reference to their degree of voluntariness. As they note, most programmes are not simply informative but often involve some element of persuasion as well. They argue that programmes should maintain, to the degree possible, options for voluntary behaviour and personal freedom on the part of the individual (Faden and Faden, 1978).

It is more likely that the classes must have overlapped and physicians must have shared the ideals and prohibitions of the hierarchical order. The place of palpation as an investigative tool is a case in point. Although palpation is an aspect of physical examination, it never becomes the instrument it could have been. The taboos against touching seem to have played a role, and even if fear of contamination is accounted for, the indigenous theory of purity and pollution must have played a major role. After all, the physician was inferior because he mingled with all sorts of people of inferior classes (Chattopadhyaya, 1977).

The process of helping involves confronting one's values with others. Often there is gap between patients or client's values and what the helper views as important, or there is a direct clash between client goals and practitioners values and culture. Clinical sociologists need to have a good understanding of their own values before they can understand the value systems of others. Hoff has pointed that it is important for the helper to 'attempt to understand' the patient or client and 'to make the patient or client feel understood'. This entails removing barriers to communication such as unwarranted assumptions and double messages that are value driven. We have personal and professional codes of ethics that spell out certain limits for what constitutes acceptable and unacceptable behaviour (Hoff, 1989).

When doctors enrolled themselves in the profession, they are bound to observe certain professional ethics and decorum. That is not for sainthood but for the upkeep of a certain code of professional conduct which was practised by seniors. This gave us the social recognition and dignity which is earned collectively. In India, no qualified doctor willing to practise ethically is going to starve. There is enough revenue generation from consultancy for everybody's need, but may be not enough to everybody's greed. The 'greed' is often perceived and firmly believed as 'need' when you actually embark upon certain ambitions of life for the sake of survival in cut-throat competition. One more building block, one more operation theatre, a CT scan machine and similar sorts, for which banks are ready to advance loans fast but also quick to retract when EMIs are delayed. The stress is passed on to the middle-class patients who might not have actually needed it at all (*The Hindu*, 2011B).

It has been argued that mainstream medical ethics is biased by the assumption of a framework in which individuals are not simply free to contact with one another to provide whatever medical treatment is demanded, subject to the ability to pay. Because a high proportion of medical care is typically provided via the welfare state, and because there are legal restrictions on what treatment may be provided and by whom, an automatic divergence may exist between the wishes of patients and the preferences of medical practitioners and other parties. Tassano has questioned the idea that beneficence might in some cases have priority over autonomy. He argues that violations of autonomy more often reflect the interests of the state or of the supplier group than those of the patient (Tassano, 1995).

In the field of medicine, basic ethical conflicts are reflected in the struggle for control over knowledge, its use or misuse by professionals and the role of the state in ensuring equity in health. As the scope of medicine expanded from clinical practice to mass interventions and the realm of public health, ethical guidelines were initially built into code of conduct for physicians, the rights of patients and informed consent (Leary, 1997).

Importance of Ethics in Society

The global medical profession has maintained simple ethical standards for more than 4,000 years. For example, the Hippocratic Oath, the prayer of Moses Maimonides, the Bible, the Holy Koran, and the Islamic legacy, as well as cultures, traditions, and social morality have shaped and guided the development of ethical standards in the medical profession. The majority of these historical documents focus on 'avoiding harm to patients' (http://www.acpmedicine.com).

Numerous indicators reflect a growing interest in ethical issues in medical and health care. For example, seldom does the popular press any longer simply report the latest biomedical development. Increasingly, media coverage includes discussion of ethical issues surrounding such developments, as has been the case with reproductive technologies such as surrogate motherhood. Moreover, professional organizations are devoting more time at their meetings and give more space in their publications to discussion of ethical issues (Gottlieb et al., 1987). As a final indicator, biomedical ethics as a discipline has expanded significantly over the past decades. A cursory review of *The Bibliography of Bioethics*, a major bibliographical resource for this field, reveals a large number of publications referred and the scope of ethical issues covered (Walters, 1975).

Against this background one might suspect an equivalent development of sociological interests in biomedical ethics. This is so because many issues in biomedical ethics are sociological topics of major interest. For example, work in the area of medical care ethics, particularly work focusing on the rights and duties of medical professionals and patients, bears directly on the evolving nature of the doctor-patient relationship (Stacey, 1985). Likewise, work in the ethics of human research focuses on such topics as investigator-subject relationships and the social control of science (Barber et al., 1973). Ethical analysis of medical and health care public policy has significant implication for such macro sociological issues as equality in access to care and the role of the professions in determining the availability of medical and health care services (Mechanic, 1979).

Ethics in Practice

Bioethicists often refer to the four basic principles of health care ethics when evaluating the merits and difficulties of medical procedures. The use of reproductive technology raises questions in each of these areas. Ideally, for a medical practice to be considered 'ethical', it must respect the five main principles of ethics which are usually considered to be:

(i) Truthfulness and confidentiality.
(ii) Autonomy.
(iii) Informed consent.
(iv) Beneficence and Nonmaleficence.
(v) Justice.

Truthfulness and Confidentiality

Truthfulness is about telling the truth to someone who has the right to know the truth. For example, if you have been informed about the result of an HIV test taken by someone in your community who then asks to know his/her result, you should tell the person the truth even though this might be very upsetting to that person. The concept of truthfulness urges the professional not to lie. On the other hand, the concept of confidentiality urges you to keep a secret by which we mean knowledge of information that a person has the right or obligation to conceal. For example, if the family of a person who has had an HIV test demands that you give them the result, you must not tell them. You must keep the result confidential unless your client gives you permission to tell his family.

Autonomy

Autonomy is another ethical principle that you may already be aware of, but not know by that name. The term refers to every individual's right to self-determination, independence and freedom to make his own choices. In the context of health care, the concept of autonomy is most concurred with the ethical obligation of the practitioner to respect their client's right to make decisions about his own health. Autonomy must be respected even if you, as the health care provider, do not agree with the client's decision. However, there are conditions in which that personal choice or autonomy may be restricted because of concern for the well-being of the community. For instance, if a communicable disease, such as tuberculosis is diagnosed, clients can be required to take prescribed medication and may have to be isolated to prevent the spread of the infection's agent to others.

Informed Consent

Informed consent means that each person who has any sort of procedure done to them in a health care context should give their approval for that procedure to be done to them. In order to be fully informed, it is the duty of the health care worker to tell the person exactly what the procedure will involve as well as the things that might happen if the procedure is not carried out.

Beneficence and Nonmaleficence

The term beneficence tells you about 'doing good' for your client, for instance by providing immunization. On the other hand, the concept of nonmaleficence tells you to 'do no harm' either intentionally or unintentionally to your clients, for instance, not abandoning a client who is in need of your services. However, there are circumstances in which, it is impossible to 'do good' and 'avoid doing harm' all at the same time. For instance, you may plan to provide birth control to all the women in your locality who are in need of it, but resource availability, cultural beliefs of the community, client's relation to the service and other factors can limit you from doing good to the greatest number. Moreover, you cannot always avoid doing harm to a client, for instance, in times when a communicable disease arises in your vicinity, you may have to suggest isolating individuals with the infection against their will to contain the spread of the disease and for good of the majority.

Justice

Justice is a complex ethical principle and it entails fairness, equality and impartiality, in other words, it is the obligation to be fair to all people. Most health practitioners will understand about justice without necessarily having come across the word itself. Suppose a health practitioner has to carry out routine antenatal care and check the pregnancy status of A's wife. The family of the health practitioner has a family dispute with A's family and she only spends few minutes with A's wife and does not tell her about all the services that are available for women when they are pregnant. Another health practitioner is working in a community which is spread out over a large rural area. The practitioner is too lazy to go to the farthest homes to incite them to participate in an environmental sanitation campaign.

IV

Ethical Theories

Ethical theories are bodies of ethical principles drawn together into a system. Four of the major ethical theories are Care Based, Communitarian, Deontology and Utilitarianism.

Ethical principles are the main foundation of ethical theories and in turn, serve as the foundation for ethical rules. Four major principles have been central to medical or health care ethics. The principle of autonomy involves a moral belief in personal freedom of will or action and respect for the self-directedness of others. A corollary principle is respect for persons. Ethically and legally, doctrines of informed consent and rights to refuse treatment are grounded in the principles of autonomy and respect for persons. The principle of beneficence and nonmaleficence are major prospects in health care. Beneficence involves positive actions to do good, to remove harmful conditions, or to seek to prevent harm. Nonmaleficence, in turn, means not inflicting harm, as expressed in a central injunction of medical ethics: 'First of all do not harm'. 'Risk benefit' analyses as well as 'due care' standards at least implicitly invoke these two ethical principles. Justice, the fourth and perhaps most complex ethical principle, involves two major subprinciples. Commutative justice focuses on the rights and duties of individuals in various relationships, especially those formed by voluntary commitments and contracts as between physician-patient, teacher-student, or lawyer-client. Distributive justice, one of the oldest and most intractable topics in philosophy, is concerned with the proper or just distribution of social benefits and burdens under conditions of scarcity. The allocation of health care resources and cost containment, two of the major preoccupations in medical care and public policy in the 1980s, depend, in part, on varying conceptions of distributive justice. Ethical rules, comprising the third level of moral discourse, often blend with ethical principles. Rules state that particular actions should or should not be taken because they are morally right or wrong. Ethical judgments and actions, finally, are based on belief about a particular situation as well as the values brought to that situation (Beauchamp and Childress, 1983). This is the 'real world' arena of applied normative ethics, in which individuals both draw upon and generate the ethical rules and principles that form ethical theories:

Care Based Theory

A type of ethical theory of health care is based on the two central constructive ideas of mutual interdependence and emotional response. The ethics of care is a rejection of impartial, principle-driven, dispassionate reasoning and judgment that has often dominated the models and paradigms of bio-ethics. Its origins are developmental, psychology, moral theory and feminist writings. Its moral concern is with needs and corresponding responsibility as they arise within a relationship. Moral response is individualized and is guided by the private norms of friendship, love and care than by abstract rights and principles.

Communitarianism Theory

Any ethical theory of health care, according to which everything fundamental in ethics drives from communal values, the common good, social goals, traditional practices and cooperative virtues. Commitment is to the general welfare to common purposes and to education of community members. Beliefs and principles, shared goals and obligations are seen as products of the communal life. Conventions, traditions and social solidarity play a prominent role in communitarianism.

Deontological Theory

Any type of ethical theory that maintains the some features of actions other than or in addition to consequences make the actions right or wrong. A major postulate is that we may not use or mistreat other people as a means to our happiness or to that of others. Deontological theories guide action with a set of moral principles or moral rules that are fundamental. Deontology judges the moral correctness of a belief or act in its own right, rather than in terms of its consequences. Thus, deontologists judge rightness or wrongness before the fact (a priori), in term of what they believe are fundamental and universally binding moral duties. This theory is sometimes called the Kantion theory because the work of Immanuel Kant (1724–1804) has a deep affect on its formulation.

Utilitarianism Theory

Utilitarianism judges the moral rightness or wrongness of an act by its non-moral consequences. Because utilitarian's think in terms of such means-to-ends moral reasoning, utilitarian ethics is especially compatible with science, medicine, and public health. Consider an action as morally right if its outcomes or consequences are good for the greatest number of population. It focuses on the greatest good for the greatest number. The theory disregards individual rights and considers the welfare of the greatest majority to be the most important factor.

After discussing the concepts and theories of health rights and ethics we will review the literature related with the health rights, medical ethics and related dimensions to health.

V

Review of Studies

Number of sociological studies have been researched on health care practices, doctor-patient communication, access to treatment and utilization of health care in public and private health facilities, preferences or choice of treatment, doctors as professional, etc. Few studies have also been done on cost of treatment, affordability, cost-benefit analysis. However, very few studies have been conducted on health rights and medical ethics. A brief overview of some of studies will be attempted here, thereby situating the ethics and health rights in the context of present study. We have categorized the studies under review in the following headings. These are as follows:

1. Studies on doctor-patient communication.
2. Studies related to the informed consent in medical practice.
3. Studies related to access to treatment and utilization of health care.
4. Studies related to cost of treatment.

5. Studies related to patient's choice of treatment and human rights.
6. Studies related to profession of medicine, medical negligence and doctors' ethics.

Studies on Doctor-Patient Communication

The interaction between doctors and patients becomes cardinal not only in the process of medical care, but also within the institution of medicine. It is through this interaction, the basic components of medical care like diagnosis, prognosis and therapeutics get accomplished. Additionally, this interaction can be seen as part of the whole process of medical care where both the actors are influenced by the changing medical knowledge. The doctors' responsibility in terms of medical ethics and patients' right to receive health care is also understood through the process of interaction.

Advani (1980) in his book *Doctor-Patient Relationship in Indian Hospitals* points out that the patients were not given sufficient attention, as the major role attributed to them was to help the physician in their maximum possible capacity in the collection of information about illness for rendering better care. Moreover, from a professional perspective, another stream of studies examined the temperament, attitude and behaviour of doctors and patients and tired to link them to the socio-economic class of the respective actors, thereby showing conflict between them.

Hasan (1979) in his study *Medical Sociology of Rural India* found out that a doctor treated the villagers with sympathy, talked to them very mildly, paid enough attention to each patient, made queries from the patient or his relatives and examined his body with hand or stethoscope. Among the qualities which the people attributed to the doctor, was his quality of paying equal attention to all without any discrimination. The doctor was devoid of casteism or communalism, made no distinction between men, women or children and did not show any favour to the rich. He paid more attention to the poor and did not charge any fees for home visits from them and sometimes he himself brought costly medicines to the poor patients and did not charge even the actual cost.

Regarding 'structural' and 'processual' analysis of the medical professionals in the hospital settings and the nature and pattern of clientele developed with the patient, Nagla (1988) mentions that the medical practitioner enjoys a respectable position in community or society. However, because of lack of facilities in the rural areas, urban orientation, living styles, etc. the medical professionals continue to work in urban areas. In order to get health medical care, people from villages have to look towards medical professionals in urban areas. In view of this, hospitals provide a good setting to study the doctor-patient relationship in the context of recruitment, socialization process of the doctors and that of expectations and satisfaction level of the patients from the doctors with whom they develop clientele for a short or long period depending upon nature of disease and severity of illness.

Social scientists like Parsons (1951), Freidson (1961) and Bloom (1963) have viewed that the mutual relationship between physician and patient is crucial in health care seeking behaviour. One dimension of this relationship, as argued by Larsen and Rootman (1976), that is of interest to both researchers and health professionals is level of patient's satisfaction with medical services. This is crucial because patient satisfaction is an important factor in health care as it influences whether a patient seeks medical help, whether he/she complies with a therapeutic regimen, and maintains a counting relationship with a physician. It is generally assumed that a patient's general level of satisfaction is influenced by a physician's role performance since a role consists of a set of behavioural expectations, which contain a normative component. In medical situation, both the patient and the physician hold different expectations.

Studies Related to the Informed Consent in Medical Practice

The doctrine of informed consent in medical practice has evolved during the past few decades. In medical context, the doctrine of informed consent implies that the person, that is, the patient, is vested with the right to decide which diagnostic and treatment procedures should be used to manage illness. His formal permission or consent is necessary before the physician undertakes his medical treatment along the lines chosen by the patient. It is legally binding on the treating doctor to inform his patient about the disease, its prognosis and the various possible lines of treatment. He must tell the patient about the different therapeutic alternatives for the treatment of his disease, the risks and side effects they carry and their expected outcomes. The consent was given in the context of an asymmetrical power relationship between the patient and doctor, wherein the former submitted to the latter's directives. As a matter of fact, it was assumed by all that having chosen his physician, the patient could just rely on the doctor of his choice for taking all the decisions on his behalf and looking after all aspects of the illness and its management to the best of his ability. In contrast to this, in the doctrine of informed consent, the emphasis is on the patient's active role in decision-making which is to be governed by principles of rationality and of equality between him and the doctor. This means that the patient should first receive all the information from the doctor and comprehend all the significant aspects of the treatment options before he takes his decision in favour of any one of them and records it in a legal language. The medical institutions also may be lacking even the basic infrastructure, tools and trained personnel to offer what the patient wants. The lag between information about options which the patient possesses and their availability is likely to create confusion, if not misunderstanding and distrust, between the doctor and the patient (Minocha, 2010).

Physician's ethical and professional obligation to provide relevant information and explanations to the patients in order to help them make up their mind about management of their aliments is not an easy task to carry out. This job is facilitated if the patients have some general knowledge about the modern system of medicine. Many Indian patients do not understand the functions of procedures such as drawing blood samples, measuring blood pressure, various invasive and non-invasive techniques and procedures, the use of anaesthesia, X-ray, ultra-sound, endoscopy, etc. The doctor would have to explain these to the ignorant patient, who may be hearing about them for the first time and does not understand how they are carried out. In other words, the doctor would have to first educate the patient about modern medicine and then inform him about particular treatment options in order to translate the doctrine of informed consent into action. This may, however, consume a lot of his professional time which he may not like (Gopal, 2004).

In his study of Indian patients, Sriram et al. (1991) noted that, in the doctor's opinion, illiteracy of the patients was the main constraint in providing information in order to obtain consent.

Evidently, in more literate societies, where people have had exposure to modern medicine for generations, the task of the doctor to inform the patient becomes easier and faster. Far from being passive recipients, the patients can critically evaluate whatever they are told and discuss their doubts with their doctors. The primary interest of the patient and his well-wishers is in his getting cured and returning to his normal routine at the earliest. The chief merit of the doctrine of informed consent is believed to be that by involving the patient in his own treatment he is given a sense of participation in the treatment process. Instead of being a passive recipient of medications, etc. the patient becomes a consciously active participant. It follows that the patient's compliance, which was presumed in the earlier paradigm, now has to be deliberately evoked by the doctor. The doctor is obliged to empower the patient by imparting information to him so that he can make well-considered rational decisions. Having done so, the patient would be able to assume responsibility for his decisions and not blame the doctor for unexpected outcomes unduly. In other words, the doctrine safeguards the interests of both.

Studies Related to Access to Treatment and Utilization of Health Care

Once with the doctor, the patient is closer to the resources that the doctor has and which the patient wants; these resources are treatment and information. Treatment is the practical application of the doctor's knowledge. Only the doctor can prescribe certain drugs, only the doctor can refer the person to hospital for treatment that he himself cannot give; only certain persons have the skill and physical equipment needed to apply the knowledge in the practical solution of problems.

In the study of medicine there has been little work on how the doctor makes treatment decisions. There are the public statements of doctors as to how diagnosis is done, and they are to be found in the literature on medical education, ideal statements about how to diagnose the problem of the patient. It is an area which has been little researched perhaps because it centres on the sensitive issue of doctor's clinical freedom. The process of consultation is very complex and the patient has to be taken into account if one wants to understand how treatment decisions are made. The patient has ways of influencing what treatment the doctor will give. His self-presentation is a strategy to influence the outcome of the consultation. In this sense, then, the outcome of the consultation is negotiable, even if the level of interaction is little overt bargaining over what the treatment will be (Stimson and Webb, 1975).

Krishnan (1994) has focused on the inter-state variation in the utilization of health services for in-patient care and has raised the important issue of the cost of treatment and the burden of treatment that fall on the lower strata of people. To him the discussion of health care financing and provision include access to health care and the quality of health services, the importance of building stocks and capital formation in health services, cost effectiveness and the role of technology in determining cost of health care.

Poverty often causes sickness and determines the disease patterns – hence the expression 'diseases of poverty'. The poor can even to some extent become biologically adapted to substandard condition of life and consider their sickness as normal. Access to health system is moreover deeply conditioned by one's possessions and income. The underlying cause of disease and health among the poor is this cruelly unequal distribution of wealth of land, of educational opportunity, of political representation and of basic human rights and this inequality is the primary disease. Though all varieties of health services are available in our cities, not all sections of the community are benefited by these facilities (Umashankar and Misra, 1993).

Sundar (1995) in her study based on National Council of Applied Economic Research (NCAER) data of 1992 revealed that the utilization of health services depends on the availability of quality health care services at a reasonable distance and on the ability of the people to utilize health services effectively. The provision of appropriate health infrastructure is a necessary but not a sufficient condition for health care utilization. A number of socio-economic factors such as financial status, caste, occupation, education and gender have great influence on the perceived need for medical care and affect the access to health care facilities. The study categorically proved that with an increase in the level of education, utilization of private health facilities goes up and the utilization of public health facilities comes down.

The utilization of government health services is very poor in India in general and particular in Kerala. The NSS and NCAER data of 1992 provides a picture of degree of health services utilization in India across three stage categories, i.e. low, medium and high expenditure group. It is found that the level of government expenditure had direct influence on the availability as well as utilization of various health services in the country. The pattern of utilization shows that public institutions are utilized more for in-patient care; and for out-patient care, majority of them prefer private doctors and private clinics. They revealed that the cost of hospital treatment in urban areas is higher compared to private sector hospitals. The study observed the growing popularity of indigenous non-allopathic systems and growth in private sectors involvement in expensive tertiary care (Purohit and Siddique, 1994).

Rao (1981) in his study *Study on Socio-economical and Demographic Correlation of Medical Care Utilization and Health Behaviour* points out that the low and very low social classes use mostly the government health services because of their poverty. They are also not aware of all the services available in General Hospitals and as a result their use is restricted to outpatient department mostly. In the caste-wise utilization of health services in India, the awareness of medical facilities is the lowest among scheduled castes and scheduled tribe groups. They prefer government hospitals; choose a place where treatment is offered free of cost and rarely go to a private practitioner.

Common complaints against public care cited in the recent NSSO (2006) and NFHS (1998–99 and 2005–06) include: 'Not satisfied with medical treatment', 'lack of availability of services', 'long waiting times', 'poor quality of care', and poor interpersonal interactions. Additionally, assessment of the public sectors underscore poor technical competence, poor accessibility to services, inadequacy of drugs and supplies, poor staff availability, and poor quality and amenities (Rao et al., 2005).

The quality of health services is dependent on a number of factors related to technical competence, accessibility to services, interpersonal relations and presence of adequate drugs, supplies, staff and facility amenities. Several studies have commented on the variable quality of public services due to lack of adequate infrastructure, human resources and indifferent behaviour of public employees (Government of India, 2006).

During the 1990s there had been stagnation in the number of rural public health institutions and beds in public hospitals. Simultaneously, there had been an increase of beds in private hospitals. The National Sample Survey data shows that respondent perceptions of not accessing care due to financial constraints increased from 10 per cent to 20 per cent in rural areas and 15 per cent to 25 per cent in urban areas from 1986 to 1996. The rate of untreated ailments increased by 40 per cent for the poorest expenditure deciles. Also, the poor still resort to the public services for most of their secondary and tertiary level care than do the better off (Iyer and Sen, 2000).

More recent surveys and studies also show that people are not satisfied with public services, and highlight the lack of infrastructure and indifferent and rude behaviour of personnel as important reasons for not using public services. According to the NSSO, 'not satisfied with medical treatment' ranks as the primary reason in both rural and urban areas. This is followed by 'lack of availability of services' in rural and 'long waiting' in urban areas. Similarly, the latest NFHS shows that the perception of 'poor quality of care' is the most important reason across selected states. The survey itself does not provide insight into what the determinants of quality are in health services, determinants of quality include clinical and interpersonal dimensions and these influence the choice and utilization of ANC (Rani et al., 2007).

The regulatory and institutional mechanisms for promoting accountability to consumers of health services are extremely weak in both the public and private sectors. Some key areas in the public sector that lack accountability are absenteeism of providers, indifferent behaviour of service providers and corruption. The private sector is prone to the overuse and misuse of technology and unethical practices and there is very little accountability. Studies have shown that there is a high rate of absenteeism among medical and paramedical personnel in the Indian health services. The absence rates are much higher in poorer areas, more among doctors than health workers and at the primary health centres as compared to the secondary or tertiary levels (Chaudhury et al., 2006).

There have been a series of studies documenting the precarious situation vis-à-vis the provision of public health facilities in India. Most of them focus on access and quality issues, which deter people from utilizing government health services. Banerjee, Deaton and Duflo (2004) have also investigated the links between non-utilization and administrative factors such as absenteeism among the health staff in the rural areas, as well as the presence of alternative informal sources of medical care. They also find instances of untrained and uninformed quacks being frequently consulted in the rural areas. Even in the fee-paying urban private sector, one particular study reports a lack of knowledge among medical practitioners in Delhi for common symptoms of diseases such as tuberculosis (Das and Hammer, 2007).

Apart from absenteeism it is well known that there is corruption in the public health services. Patients report of corruption in terms of bribes demanded for admission and treatment in public institutions. Corruption is also rife in recruitment, promotion and transfer of personnel; admission to medical and paramedical education; procurement of drugs and technology (Sakthivel, 2005). Corruption is not restricted to the public sector alone. The private sector also has its share of corruption in the form of unethical practices. There is a well-worked out system of paying commissions when doctors refer patients for diagnostic testing in the private sector. Similarly, the pharmaceutical industry through their representatives offers a variety of incentives to doctors for prescribing specific brands of medicines (Baru, 1998; Phadke, 1998). With liberalization and increase in public subsidies to the private sector and to the tertiary sectors, there are reports of non-compliance to the equity conditionality by corporate hospitals.

Another reason for the displacement of the poor from public sector provision is the introduction of user fees. The argument that such fees generate resources from those who can pay to improve the quality of care for those who cannot has been proven wrong. Not only do they squeeze the non-paying poor out of public hospitals, but the upper middle class has stopped using these financially constrained hospitals. Thus, articulate voices that could protest against and resist dwindling quality are lost. Even if a hospital somehow manages to improve its services, it fails to improve the system as a whole since there is no mechanism of risk pooling. Together, the general policy of tax reduction and the introduction of user fees shift the burden of hospital costs on to the poor, who suffer a greater burden of sickness owing to poverty, greater exposure to risk and lack of basic services. The rich thus benefit from the current reforms at the expense of the poor (Krishnan, 1999).

Popular discussions around the performance of a government are usually not cast in quantitative terms. Much more typical is the impressionistic argument based on certain cases one happens to know of. Even when certain numbers are used they are almost invariably selectively picked up to support one's predetermined position. In West Bengal, it is often argued by the government-side that in spite of all the alleged ills of the government hospitals, more than 80 per cent of all the patients in West Bengal go to them for treatment. The elementary distinction that one has to make here is the one between in-patient and out-patient care services. While around 80 per cent of the in-patient cases are treated in government hospitals only 14 per cent of the out-patient cases are treated in government facilities. High percentage of out-patient cases going to private facilities is taken as indicative of the failure of the health system. As far as the out-patient services are concerned, people are clearly exercising their exit option, and we find nothing unusual about West Bengal, given the experience of the rest of India as well as many other countries (Chakraborty and Mukherjee, 2003).

Bhatnagar et al. (1988) in his slum study revealed the high utilization of private sources of health services by the urban dwellers in Delhi. It shows that 62 per cent use purely private sources, 24 per cent both government and private and only 14 per cent used government sources alone indicating the sad state of affairs of the government health centres and the need for improving the accessibility and utilization of government health centres.

In India, the private sector consists of a small but powerful corporate sector, a rapidly proliferating set of nursing homes, and a vast body of private practitioners ranging from specialists to untrained individuals. The professionals view the latter with contempt and their practice is in the process of being banned, even though they are often the only healers available for the poor. The schemes set in place to upgrade and train these practitioners have been severely criticized by professional doctors. Similarly, the nursing homes are a mixed bag of doubtful quality providers, as revealed by the qualifications of their personnel and the quality of their infrastructure (Baru, 1998).

The inability of the state to rationalize, control or monitor the private sector is one of the outcomes of the current strategy of decontrol and of building partnerships and social contracts with the private sector. The hold of the private sector on medical care is thus rising and significant and in our view, endangering whatever remains of primary health care. This uncontrolled expansion has led to growing malpractice in the illegal sale of body parts such as kidneys, human experiments without informed consent and sale of dangerous contraceptives through the private sector. The private sector, therefore, is highly prone to providing declining quality without adequate checks and safeguards (VAHAI, 1993).

The assumption that private services offer superior quality of services is not adequately supported by any hard evidence. While some private sector facilities offer good quality services, this cannot be generalized because of the heterogeneity of facilities, personnel and their practices. Evidence from micro studies is revealing. Private care practitioners along with public care practitioners, for example, in Delhi, are more skilled and knowledgeable in the wealthier areas in comparison to the poorer area (Das and Hammer, 2007).

Yesudian (1981) studied the health behaviour of four social classes – high, middle, low and very low in the utilization of health services in Bombay (now Mumbai) city. He observed that as the low and very low social class households are educationally backward, their knowledge, level of diseases, available health services, and their perception, desire to seek health services are found to be lower than that of middle and high class households.

The private sector is also gigantic but restricted to medical care, providing 80 per cent of outdoor consultations and 55 per cent of indoor care. This unregulated private sector includes a range of service providers – the non-formal practitioner, the general practitioner formally trained in modern medicine, the nursing homes and polyclinics with groups of doctor-proprietors and the hospitals with small or big corporate structure (Ashraf and Rodrigues, 2002).

Problems in the formal private sector include the following: physicians tend to over-prescribe care according to patients' ability to pay; a lack of registration procedures; badly kept records; and inadequate infrastructure with poorly trained physicians and nurses (Nandraj and Duggal, 1997). A commonly observed phenomenon is over-prescription of medicines, diagnostic testing and surgeries. Studies on informal practitioners in rural and urban areas show that they often lack qualifications and adopt irrational practices in prescribing medicines for the treatment of common illnesses. While the lack of accountability of the public sector is well known, the private sector is not any different. If anything, there are fewer checks on their accountability due to weak regulation. The role of consumer groups in ensuring accountability has been limited. An example of an effective campaign by consumer groups was when they drew attention to the rise in reported cases of medical negligence in the private sector. A few cases were registered with the consumer courts and compensation was given for medical negligence in the private sector. Since dual public and private practices are permitted, the public sector acts, at times, only as a referral portal for the legalized private practices.

Studies Related with Cost of Treatment

On the basis of literature related to comparative costs, including cost analysis of various types of services or programmes, an attempt has been made here to make a brief review of the important works among them.

The cost of treatment consists of doctors fees, cost of medicine, hospital charges, laboratory charges, transport cost to access the medical facility, wages and income lost during the period of disease, etc. Here costs are classified into direct cost and indirect cost. Direct cost consists of consultation fee, cost of medicine, hospital rent, charges for lab tests, etc. On the other hand, indirect cost consists of travelling expenses of the patient and accompanying persons, food and accommodation of the companion, wages and income loss due to illness, etc.

The main objective of the Babson's study on 'Disease Costing, Studies in Social Administration' is to drive a methodology for costing treatments. The study has outlined in considerable detail the methods of attributing hospital resources to treatments in the given disease categories. Market values are used to estimate costs. The author argues that the study justifies considerable optimism regarding the feasibility of disease costing (Babson, 1973).

According to Reddy (1995) improved health contributes to economic growth in four ways; it reduces production loss caused by workers' illness; it permits the use of natural resources that had been nearly inaccessible because of disease; it increases the enrolment of children in school and it frees for alternative use of recourses that would otherwise have to spent on treating illness.

The burden of disease in terms of the number of days lost due to illness and the costs incurred by the household, through cost of treatment and through loss of household income. The study concludes that allopathy is the preferred system of medicine, acute morbidity is the major cause in the total number of days of work lost and that the average cost of treatment of acute illness is high (Krishnaswami, 2004).

The average direct cost of treatment regarding acute illness as well as chronic illness under all the system of medicine in urban areas is greater than that in rural areas. In rural areas the average direct cost of treatment under allopathy for acute illness is greater than the average direct cost of chronic illness. There are variations in the preference pattern of the people for different system of medicine in rural and urban areas. The preference for the allopathy and ayurveda is greater in urban areas while the preference for homoeopathy is relatively more in rural areas. There is high rural-urban disparity in the availability of and accessibility to different systems of medicine (Anitha, 2011).

The benefits and costs arising from the treatment of rheumatic diseases have been dealt in Brooks' analysis. The costs considered are the costs of providing hospital and other facilities for treatment. The benefits are those arising from the productive output gained from patients who are able to return to work. The study assumes that all the improvements in health are due to the treatment. The costs of treatment are estimated using market values. The value of the production of those in employment is valued at gross earnings. A wage is computed for housewives using the wage of domestic helps. The study concludes that there is a prima facie case for the investment of resources in centres of rheumatic diseases (Brooks, 1969).

The main purpose of Cooper and Rice's study on 'The Economic Cost of Illness Revisited' was to indicate the costs to society for different forms of illnesses. The economic cost of illness was considered to be due to the direct resource outlays for prevention, detection and treatment and the indirect costs or loss in output due to disability and premature death. The cost of pain and suffering were noted but not considered. Aggregate data from a number of sources were used for treatment. They found that the total cost of illness for 1972 was US $ 189 billion at a 4 per cent discount rate. About $ 40 billion was for persons suffering from diseases related to the circulatory system, $ 27 billion for accident victims and $ 17 billion each for cancer patients and victims of gastro diseases (Cooper and Rice, 1976).

The high costs of curative medicine in both the private and public sector discriminate against the poor. Those in greatest need can least afford to pay for expensive treatment and to bear the costs of travel to urban hospitals; this accounts partly for the underutilization of medical services reported in several studies. The introduction of health insurance has resulted also in lower standards of service to the poor and especially rural people who are excluded from these schemes. But the taxes of the poor are used to finance curative medicine and to subsidize the costs of private treatment for the few (Abel-Smith, 1976).

Rising health costs is currently a serious health financing problem. This is equally faced by developing and developed countries and all population groups. This problem arises out of various situations like rapidly rising cost of living. Also it is a by-product of rising rates of health care utilization and expansion of social security measures by welfare governments in developing countries. The medical technologies have also contributed to the rising cost of health care. The solution lies in the measures through appropriate technologies and interventions (Goel, 2002).

Studies Related with Patients Choice of Treatment and Health Rights

The primary target in quality of life concerns, as they relate to health care, is most often the patient, of course. However, for the purpose of making quality of life assessments, significant others in the life of the patients should often be the focus of evolution as well. For example, in the case of the patient with severe Alzheimer's diseases, the health care concerns appropriately centre first on the patient. However, in terms of quality of problems, the family of the patient can be even more profoundly affected by Alzheimer than the patient, who may be in a sense 'lost' or impervious in the dementia of the illness.

It will be assumed for the purposes of the description of the consultation process that the person has come to see consultation with the doctor as appropriate for their problem. This may not be an easy decision to reach. It is often difficult to identify and categorize problems that may be illness. There is usually some uncertainty in the person's mind. People do not always know whether they are ill or not, or whether they are ill enough to take some action about the illness.

It is estimated that American presently suffering some degree of dementia, there may be up to three times that number of close family members whose lives are deeply affected by the emotional, physical, social and financial burdens caring for Alzheimer's victims. The needs of an ill or frail parent with Alzheimer's disease may create or exacerbate a condition of multiple demands for their children's time, energy, money and emotional support, resulting in increased health problems for care givers (Weiler, 1987).

Given the impact of the diseases of the Alzheimer's patients on their own quality of life, family members may respond with depression, resentment, frustration and in other ways that can affect how they provide care for the patient. Thus, the impact of Alzheimer's disease on the family as well as the patient may have powerful implications for planning treatment programmes and for providing continued support from family care givers (Zarit et al., 1985).

Impingement of quality of life issues on the family are dramatically illustrated as well, in the case of the dying patient. In this instance can we consider that the whole family is also the 'patient' in a sense? In the case of the terminal patient, studies have shown that the progress of bereavement in family members may be ongoing before death has occurred, that while the patient is still present to interact with the grieving person. Feelings of sorrow, hostility and resentment towards the dying person for leaving may be present before death has occurred. If the terminal illness is one that can be interpreted as preventable as in the case of the patient dying of lung cancer, feelings of resentment toward the patient may complicate the life of the patient's family. In the case of some family members, such as young children of the dying person the emotional burden of the dying process may be especially hard (Levine and Scotch, 1970).

It is known from quantitative studies on patient's use of prescribed medicines, that a high portion of patients do not follow the instructions of their doctors. If the treatment is a drug, the patient may decide not to take the prescription to the chemist or may have it dispensed and not use the drug and then discontinue, or may begin to use the drug and then discontinue, or may use it with a frequency or in a dosage other than those suggested by the doctor. Some patients do not attend hospital departments to which they have been referred by their doctors (Nuffield Provincial Hospitals Trust, 1965).

Making man and women aware of their rights towards good sanitation and health is also likely to boost other sectors as well. To make this point more clear, let me take the example of access to unmet need. Meeting the unmet need for contraceptives will not only help in arresting the population growth, but also will help in deriving a number of other benefits including overall health gains. Study has demonstrated that if we meet the unmet need in the next five years, we are likely to save nearly 1,50,000 mothers from dying during pregnancy, delivery or within 42 days of delivery. Increased survival of mothers will in turn improve the survival of a large number of children during their first year of life, many of whom would have otherwise died. Moreover, meeting the needs could further reduce the number of women who seek services to abort unwanted pregnancies, many of whom opt for unsafe and illegal abortions. In addition to fulfilling the rights of women and men, we are also likely to save more than ₹ 4,000 millions in the next five years which will be otherwise spent on providing abortion and maternal care services (Ram, 2011).

Banerji (1982) points out in his study that doctors do not behave in the same manner towards all patients for medical check-ups. Patients with resistance and those who need the new drug regime the most, may not get it. This denies the right of individuals to quality treatment.

In instances where a chronic or terminal illness or injury bears some stigma, such as the sequel of suicide, AIDS, self-caused injuries from drunken driving, or use of illegal drugs, the quality of life of family members may be negatively affected both immediately and over the long term (Kane et al., 1985). Beyond the perspective on physical loss of the patient, there may be problem of medical care expenses, depleted finances, loss of income from the wage earner, the need for adjustment of role relations and responsibilities and the loss of the emotional and affection support from the patient. Although many of these qualities of life, problems of the family are inherent problem of life, some of them may be profitably mediated by the physician or by administrative polices of health care organizations (Croog and Levine, 1982).

If the quality of life of the family as well as the patient indeed can be defined as a legitimate of the object concern, this has implications for changes in the provision of counselling and social services, the behaviour of physicians and other health care personnel and administrative polices of health care organizations. Many of the problems may be more effectively ameliorated by their interventions. Although programmes and polices of many professions and organizations within the health care system are already in place and are proceeding along these lines, there is continuing controversy about their relative importance and their financial costs, given other priorities for the care of patients.

In the case of cancer, the problem of patient choices of treatment has been a continuing theme, and the popular culture has disseminated information about a variety of alternatives. The treatment of some cancer patients has been complicated by the lure of non-traditional health practitioners and health interventions. This has been in part a reaction to observations that some traditional medical and surgical approaches are painful, do not appreciably extend survival time, and have undesirable consequences regarding quality of life. Hence, patients have sought out chiropractors, naturopaths, acupuncturists, spiritual healers, nutrition therapists, and other nonmedical practitioners (Silberfarb et al., 1980).

The right to autonomous decision-making is not universally available, due to economic and social realities. A core ethical principle should be applied equitably to all patients. This presumes that all patients have equal access to all medical options. The world is not ideal, however, and many patients' options are limited by socio-cultural boundaries to medical care or the availability of funding to pay for medical care. It is absurd to say that such patients have a choice, when limited choices are available to them. For women with limited access to the full spectrum of health care services, the principle of autonomy is of very limited value as a guiding principle in making medical decisions (Hedgecoe, 2006).

Studies Related with Profession of Medicine, Medical Negligence and Doctors' Ethics

The medical profession is often held to represent the professional ideal in modern society. It ranks high in social prestige and financial remuneration and it performs essential services within the community backed by specialized and effective knowledge and expertise. Doctors occupy a higher social status in the society not only because of high professionalization but also because they deal with health and life of human beings (Elliot, 1972).

It has often been claimed that our society, as perhaps most, is more enamoured with medical intervention to correct health problems than it is with preventing the health problems in the first place. This ready acceptance or desire for curative intervention rather than preventive maintenance has been fuelled by a long list of biomedical and scientific breakthroughs that have contributed to the belief that, regardless of the problem, medical science can be counted on to produce a quick fix, such as a vaccine or a cure.

The recognition that an individual's behaviour can contribute significantly to the risk of premature morbidity or mortality has led to numerous admonitions, on the one hand, for individuals to be more responsible for their own health and discussions, on the other hand, of the right of the state to develop policies that coerce individuals to lead more healthy or risk-reducing lives (Knowles, 1977).

In an ethical analysis of the responsibility of the state and the right of the individual concerning health, Wikler (1978) has examined three ethical justifications for state-initiated programmes in health promotion that may not correspond to individual preference profiles regarding behaviours or lifestyles. The first justification is based on the notion that health is a valued good. It may not be a terminal or ultimate value in most individuals' lives, but clearly many normal and routine life events cannot be experienced without a modicum of health. Accordingly, Wikler argues that state initiated health promotion programmes could be justified ethically on the basis of the principle of beneficence, or doing well. In pointing this out, Wikler also notes that health promotion programmes run into problems of possible charges of paternalism, that is forcing individuals to do something that, while it may be in the individuals long-term health interest, is something the individual may not want to do in the short run. Potential infringement on individual liberty is a major ethical dilemma in virtually any health promotion programme that goes beyond the simple provision of information. A second ethical premise examined to justify state-based health promotion initiatives rests on the argument that it is unfair for some individuals to act as they please when such action leads to significant burdens on society. A third principle Wikler identifies is that of promoting the general societal welfare. The argument here is that the state has a right to promote the general welfare, because this leads to improved societal productivity, a better economy and so forth. The latter are goods that can benefit a majority of individuals in a society. Such benefits may be used to justify curtailment of individual lifestyle of those persons who engage in high-risk behaviours.

In one of his study related to 'Rural Elderly: Health Status and Available Health Services', Kumar (1996) described that much of the disability and ill health of old people is the result of medical negligence. The medical profession is beginning to realize that old people do respond to treatment and can recover to function to a surprising degree. It is observed that though majority of the elderly need medical aid for longer period from government hospitals, they are not able to visit the hospitals on account of long distance and poor transportation facilities, and lack of personal help. Poverty is also one of the important factors, preventing the elderly to avail proper medical aid. Like children, the aged too need health and personal care and hence there is need to establish separate geriatric wards in the hospitals with geriatric professionals. Thus, quality of life plays a major and particularly obvious role in the treatment and control of hypertension. In its mild to moderate form this disease is virtually symptoms, but the medications can produce many side-effects, affecting quality of life and leading to noncompliance. These problems can perhaps best be addressed in clinical practice if proper inquiries are made by medical personnel and treatment is adjusted accordingly and as needed.

Certain types of people, such as students and others who are relatively mobile, are very likely to receive medical information from several doctors about the same condition, without these doctors necessarily knowing that the person has already received advice elsewhere.

If the patient is referred for an opinion, the specialists reply is sent in a letter to the first doctor and will rarely be seen by the patient. However, the specialist may be willing, or may unwittingly, divulge information that the general practitioner has not disclosed to the patient. The way he is examined, or the questions that are asked, may also help 'to give the game away' to the patient.

Doctors appear to feel the need to guard against patients 'devious' way of gaining access to information. Very often the patient's strategy may be met by a counter-strategy. Balint warns doctors of some patients' 'ability to play off' one doctor against another and suggests ways of combating this – by improving communications and history-taking on the part of the medical staff to prevent the patient from taking advantage of the loopholes in the system (Balint, 1971).

The issue about the 'patient's voice' does not, however, go away. This is due to changes in how people think about their health, about living with serious illness and about professional expertise. This is a continuation of the relationship of medicine to society, one that goes back to the end of the 18th century. The introduction of the new clinical techniques changed 'being a patient' from a question of how to die with contrition to one of how to survive with medical help, and ultimately how to live. In the last half century the development of new procedures such as endoscopy, of new drug therapies and recently the promise of genetic engineering not only enable survival but provoke questions of how to live when cure is not possible. The growth in the number of self-help and support groups relating to specific diseases, together with the spread of the internet and the information revolution, means that this is no longer just a practical matter (how do I survive?) but an ethical issue (how should I live my life?). The emergence of an ethics of illness means that the voice of the patient is no longer framed solely within the consulting room or the clinic. It is not something to be heard only in response to the ministrations of the doctor, but is an active part of people's use of medical help in a world where they wish to determine their own way of life (Herzlich and Pierret, 1987).

Auxiliaries, known also as dispensers, health aides and medical assistants, have been employed in some developing countries for many years but, as Djukanovic and Mach (1975) pointed out, they have been used very ineffectively in the past. Many have been underutilized, undertaking only the simplest tasks. This is partly because of opposition from the medical profession, which has claimed that it is both unethical and dangerous to entrust the care of sick people to these workers, and in several developing countries where training centres for auxiliaries existed before independence they were closed after medical schools were established. In many cases, they have been sent to the rural areas without adequate support, drugs and other resources; dissatisfaction has been reported because of low salaries, poor promotion prospects, inadequate transport and unsatisfactory living conditions. Some have been accused of treating those who pay private fees in addition to government charges and in some cases auxiliaries have left government service to establish private practices or to work for physicians in urban areas.

2

Methodology

Field and Planning of Study

Formulation of Problem

Human life is precious and every person has a fundamental right to live with dignity. It is the duty of a welfare state to protect and develop the life of every citizen and to promote his rights to health and medical care. Right to medical care is important because it relates to the very existence of human life. Medical care is as essential as the other basic needs of a person like food, water, shelter and clothing. Every nation has evolved its own system of laws to ensure the health rights of its citizens. These laws aim to establish a human system of health care based on the principles of equity, justice and efficiency. By emphasizing the rights of the citizens for proper health care, every good government tries to enhance the welfare of its people so that they can live healthy and productive lives.

Rapid developments in the medical field in the last century have revolutionized the field of medical practice. It is now possible to diagnose diseases faster and more accurately using advanced diagnostic techniques. Medical management has become more effective with referred indications having more specific action and lower side effects. Surgical treatments move towards less invasive modes of management with lesser morbidity and faster recovery. Among all these developments, the medical profession in India is at crossroad facing many ethical and health right challenges in the practice of profession. The medical fraternity is becoming more and more dependent on technology and market forces which tend to influence decision-making of doctors. The fundamental values of medicine insist that doctor's obligation is to keep the patients interests above everything else.

The important issues of autonomy, confidentiality, justice, beneficence and non-maleficence are key factors that should guide the daily decision-making by the doctor. These decisions may be involving a simple choice of antibiotics for an infection on the best medication for hypertension. It becomes more complex involving major ethical concerns in organ transplantation, clinical trials, genetic manipulation, end of life issues, or assisted reproductive techniques. However, the principle ethics remain the same for the entire above situation. The ethical guideline of medical practice provided by the Indian Medical Council (Professional Conduct, Etiquette, and Ethics Regulation, 2002) is aimed at strengthening the ethical standard among registered medical practitioners in India.

It is imperative that the present-day medical doctor have a continuing medico-legal education. Doctors have legal duty to comply with the applicable ethical regulations in their daily practice. Not conferring to ethics will be detrimental to the patient's suffering. Since patients are increasingly aware of their health rights therefore, doctors have to be conversant with basic ethical issues involved in medical practice.

The right to health is one of the economic, social and cultural human rights that requires affirmative government action to create better conditions for people rather than just governmental restraint vis-à-vis citizens. Health and human rights have explicit intrinsic connections and have emerged as powerful concepts within the rights-based approach especially so in the backdrop of weakening public health system, unregulated growth of the private sector and restricted access to health care systems leading to a accessibility of universal and comprehensive health care. A rights-based approach uses International Human Rights treaties and norms to hold governments accountable for their obligations under the treaties. It recognizes the fact that the right to health is a fundamental right of every human being and it implies the enjoyment of the highest attainable standard of health. Government has responsibility for the health of their people which can be fulfilled only through the provision of adequate health and social measures. It gets integrated into research, advocacy strategies and tools, including monitoring; community education and mobilization; litigation and policy formulation. Right to the highest attainable standard is encapsulated in Article 12 of the International Covenant on Economic, Social and Cultural Rights. It covers the underlying preconditions necessary for health and also the provisions of medical care. The critical component within the right to health philosophy is its realization.

The progressive weakening of public health systems, the growing privatization of health care and the erosion of universal access to health care are worldwide phenomena. The health sector globally is still dominated by vertical and ethnocentric approaches, often supported by 'public-private partnerships' active at several levels. There is need to replace this dominant discourse by a process aimed at universally achieving the 'right to health and to health care' as the main objective.

For a patient, the doctor is like God. And, the God is infallible. But that is what the patient thinks. In reality, doctors are human beings. And, to err is human. Doctors may commit a mistake. Doctors may be negligent. The support staff may be careless. The act of negligence may give rise to a much bigger problem. It may be due to gross negligence. Anything is possible. In such a scenario, it is critical to determine who is negligent, and under what circumstances.

An eminent English radiologist Robert Hutchison prayed: 'From ... too much zeal for the new, and contempt for the old; from putting knowledge before wisdom; science before art; cleverness before commonsense; from treating patients as cases and for making cure of disease more grievous than the endurance thereof: good Lord deliver us'. Ethics of the doctors are not good as per their duty or humanity. Very few doctors pay adequate attention towards the problem of the patient in their duty time. If anyone needs the medical help after their duty, very few of them provide their service to them; some of them may ignore or demand pay. All these show the lack of moral values or ethics (*The Times of India*, 2004).

As the scope of medicine expanded from clinical practice to mass interventions and realm of public health, ethical guidelines are very important for the code of conduct for physicians, the rights of patients and informed consent. Ethical analysis of medical health care has significant implication for issues like equality in access to care and role of medical profession in determining the availability of medical and health care services. Recently the ethical guidelines provided by Indian Medical Council 'Regulation 2002', aimed to improve the functioning of medical profession as emerging concern of organ transplantation, clinical trials, genetic manipulation, etc. has come into being. At the same time, health rights are also asserted by the patients for being more educated and with the global exposure. Thus, it becomes relevant to understand the health rights and medical ethics in the context of doctors and users of health services, i.e. patients.

Thus, in our study we set out the following objectives:

Objectives of the Study

(i) To identify the socio-economic background of doctors and indoor patients.
(ii) To understand the meaning of health, health rights and medical ethics.
(iii) To comprehend the knowledge of the patients regarding their health rights.
(iv) To analyse the knowledge and practice of doctors regarding the medical ethics.
(v) To analyse the incidents of violation of health rights as experienced by the patients and doctors.

II

Methodology

Field of the Study

Haryana is the 16th largest state in India. It came into existence on 1 November 1966 as a newly created state, carved out of the Punjab state on the basis of language. Haryana has 21 districts, 106 towns and 6,955 villages. The total population of this state, as per the report published after Census 2011, is 25, 353, 081 with a population density of 573.4 per sq km. Haryana has a very fertile land and is called the Green Land of India. The state is bordered by Uttar Pradesh in east, Punjab in west, Himachal Pradesh in north and Rajasthan in south. Union Territory of Delhi is landlocked on three sides by Haryana. Haryana is selected for the present study. This state is selected for two reasons. First, there has been a rapid economic growth in Haryana since the introduction of the Green Revolution in the 1960s. In 1981, out of the total: 99.6 per cent and 55 per cent of villages of Haryana have electricity and transport services, respectively. Male and female projected life expectancy (2011–15) rates in the state are 68.9 and 71.3 respectively against 67.3 and 69.6 years for the country (DGHS, 2014). Second, despite improvement in life expectancy and economic growth, a large number of women, i.e. 56.5 ever married women between the age-group of 15–49 are anaemic (IIPS and Macro International, 2008). Since the inception of Haryana State in 1966, there has been a significant increase in the number of health services over a period of almost four decades. Per capita expenditure on health has increased from 1.92 in 1966–67 to ₹ 734 in 2013–14. Annual growth in health expenditure is more than 15 per cent per annum from 1980–81 to 1985–86, falling to less than 5 per cent during the 1985–86 and 1990–91 and less than 10 per cent from 1990–91 to 1995–96.

Table 2.1

Health Data in Haryana

Particulars			*Numbers*
Hospitals			56
Community Health Centres			109
Primary Health Centres			357
Dispensaries/Polyclinics/Urban Health Centre			63
Urban Health Posts			16
Postpartum Centres			37
District T.B. Centres/Clinics			15
Subcentres			2,630
	Patients Treated During		
Patients	*2010*	*2011*	*2012*
Outdoor	1,89,55,488	1,66,22,780	1,67,22,218
Indoor	18,01,813	13,90,974	13,96,426
Beds Per Thousand Population			0.39
Population Served Per Medical Institution			7,980
Nurse: Bed Ratio			1:7
Doctor: Bed Ratio			1:4

Source: Director General, Health Services 2012–2013, Haryana, Panchkula, 2014.

The number of CHCs, PHCs and Subcentres and trained doctors, and paramedical personnel increased substantially in

Haryana over the last four decades. The number of doctors, nurses and paramedical staff in government health care facility and private health has also increased.

Profile of Bhiwani District

Bhiwani District is one of the largest of the 21 districts of Haryana state. Bhiwani District was created on 22 December 1972. The Bhiwani District is surrounded by Hissar District on its North, some area of Jhunjunu and Churu District of Rajasthan on its West, Mahendergarh and Jhunjunu District on its South and District Rohtak on its East.

The district occupies an area of 5,140 square kilometres (1,980 sq mi), and is situated between 28.19 degree and 29.05 degree north latitudes and 75.26 degree and 76.28 degree east longitudes. It has 442 villages, 6 Tehsil and 3 Sub-Tehsil which has a population of 1,634,445 of which male and female were 866,672 and 767,773 respectively. Average literacy rate of Bhiwani is 75.21 per cent. Gender-wise, male and female literacy is 85.65 and 63.54 respectively. Sex ratio in Bhiwani, is 886 per 1,000 male (Census, 2011). The district headquarters is the city of Bhiwani, which is around 124 kilometres from Delhi and 285 km from Chandigarh. Other major towns in the district are Siwani, Charkhi Dadri, Loharu, Tosham and Bawani Khera.

In Bhiwani District, there are 6 general hospitals, 9 CHCs, 32 PHCs and 214 SHCs (see Table 2.2).

Table 2.2

Health Infrastructure in Bhiwani District

Sr. No.	*Health infrastructure*	*Numbers*
1.	General Hospital	6
2.	Community Health Centre	9
3.	Primary Health Centre	33
4.	Subcentre	214

Source: District Statistical Department Bhiwani, 2014.

Health Institutions are providing following health services to the public through subcentres, PHC/CHC and District Hospital:

1. Primary Health Care to the patients.
2. Antenatal, Natal, Postnatal Care and Newborn Care.
3. Immunization Services on Wednesday at village level.

4. Nutrition supplements to anaemic and pregnant mothers.
5. Twenty four hours free delivery services at PHC/CHC/ District Hospital level.
6. Emergency Care at PHC level.
7. Direct Observed Treatment Short Course (DOTS) facility at subcentre level.
8. Awareness Malaria Control programme.
9. School health check-up.
10. Control of blindness.
11. Awareness regarding AIDS.

III

Sample Method

The purpose of our study is to understand the meaning of health, health rights and medical ethics, therefore, hospital institutions are taken into account. Hospitals are comprised of doctors, patients and other paramedical staff. Out of the 21 districts, we randomly selected the Bhiwani District, which is one of the largest districts in the state of Haryana. To select the hospitals for the study purpose, we decided to study both government and private hospitals in Bhiwani city. Bhiwani city is purposively selected because of presence of enough number of private hospitals where large numbers of patients seek their treatment. City of Bhiwani has one big government hospital with 22 doctors. It was established in 1976 and approximately 700–800 patients visit in a day in the Out Patient Department (OPD) and 80–90 (per day) patients in indoor. On the other hand, there are 46 well established private clinics/nursing homes/hospitals.

Out of 46 private clinics/nursing homes/hospitals, 28 are having only one doctor, 12 are having one male and one female doctor and 11 are having three or more male and female doctors. Six are only dental clinics and three are eye clinics and thirty-three private clinics/nursing homes/hospitals are providing 24 hour medical facilities. Only ten out of 46 private clinics/ nursing homes/hospitals are providing specialized facilities like maternity and childcare and five are providing treatment to children only. Among 46 private hospitals, only 2 clinics are providing emergency ambulance services, and they are J.B. Gupta Hospital and Chugh Multispecialty Hospital.

Three hospitals are providing free OPD service, which are newly established and providing free OPD facility for their advertisement and initial reputation. The oldest hospital is 'Ganpatrai Maternity and General Hospital (estab., 1954) which is run by a trust. The per day indoor patients in Ganpatrai Maternal and General Hospital are less as compared to the second oldest 'Chugh Multispecialty Hospital (estab., 1979), therefore, we selected the hospital which is the oldest in terms of year of its establishment and simultaneously has highest number of indoor patients (see Table 2.3)

For the present study, General Hospital is selected for the study purpose in the government hospital category. It has 22 doctors and 80–90 patients (per day) are treated in different indoor wards. One private hospital is selected on the basis of date of establishment and its large size in terms of indoor facility for patients. Among the list of 46 hospitals/clinic/nursing homes, Chugh hospital was selected because it was established in 1979 and it is the oldest among the private hospitals. It also has the larger number of patients in indoor facility, i.e. 10–12 patients per day in the ward.

All the doctors of selected private hospital and government hospital during the specific period, i.e. from October 2013 to December 2013 are interviewed. The patients who are having their stay in the indoor ward for more than three days are selected and interviewed. While selecting General Hospital and Chugh Private Hospital, our aim is to study hospital's functioning in the government and private settings. Government and private hospitals are chosen in order to observe the difference between the government and the private hospital services. We decided to interview all the twenty-two doctors from government hospital and all the nine doctors from Chugh Private Hospital. During the process of our interview, six doctors from the government hospital could not be interviewed as they are on long leave and from the same hospital another three doctors refused to give interview. Therefore, effectively, we interviewed thirteen doctors from government hospital and all nine doctors from Chug Private Hospital.

Patients coming to indoor clinic of hospital comprised the sample. Samples are selected to gather information about the population from which they are drawn. Sometimes it is impossible

Table 2.3

Hospital/Nursing Homes/Maternity Homes in Bhiwani City

Sr. No.	Name and year of establishment	No. of Doctors		Timing	OPD Daily	Indoor Daily	Total Bed	OPD Fee	Emergency Fee	Bed Charge Per Day
		M	F							
1.	General Hospital (1976)	13	9	24x7	700–800	80–90	300	5	5	250
2.	Panwar Maternity and Children Hospital (2011)	1	2	24x7	35–40	3–4	17	100	200	400–700
3.	Jangra Hospital and Maternity Centre (2009)	2	1	24x7	25–30	4–5	10	30	100	200–400
4.	Girdhar Hospital (2008)	1	1	Day	35–40	Nill	4	150	300	—
5.	Inderjeet Hospital (1999)	1	—	24x7	30–35	5–7	15	100	200	500–800
6.	K.M. Hospital (2006)	1	—	24x7	50–60	8–10	12	80	150	300–500
7.	Ansh Hospital (2012)	1	—	24x7	30	4–5	6	Free	100	150
8.	Prakash Dental Clinic (2013)	1	1	Day	6–10	Nill	—	30	—	—
9.	Shri Bala ji Nursing Home (2013)	1	—	24x7	15	2	3	Free	Free	Free
10	Yadav Child Hospital (2008)	1	—	24x7	110–120	2–3	16	100	200	600–1,000
11.	Verma Child Hospital (2008)	1	1	24x7	20	5–6	12	100	200	400–600
12.	Eye Q Super Speciality Hospital (2013)	2	—	Day	100–120	Nill	—	100	200	—
13.	Vandna Maternity Hospital (1992)	1	1	24x7	35–40	5–6	16	150	300	400–600
14.	Khasa Child Hospital (1995)	1	—	24x7	60–65	5–6	17	150	300	700–1,000
15.	Goyal Dental Hospital (2010)	1	1	Day	18–20	—	—	100	150	—
16.	Guliya Nursing Home (1999)	1	1	24x7	40–45	5–6	18	80	150	500–700
17.	Narendra Nateraliya (2006)	1	—	Day	60–70	Nill	6	100	—	—

Cont'd ...

... *Cont'd*

18. Sharma Hospital (2001)	1	1	24x7	20–25	5–7	16	50	100	400–500
19. City Nursing Home (1991)	1	—	24x7	40–50	5–6	19	100	200	300–600
20. Trivani Dental Hospital (2008)	1	2	Day	40–45	Nill	—	50	—	—
21. Deswal Maternity Hospital (2008)	—	1	24x7	10–15	Nill	7	50	—	—
22. J.B. Gupta Hospital (2000)	5	1	24x7	50–55	8–10	40	150	250	600–1,500
23. Prem Hospital (2000)	1	—	24x7	15–16	1–2	10	100	200	400
24. Anil Hospital (2006)	1	1	24x7	20–25	2–3	13	50	100	400–600
25. Chugh Multispecialty Hospital (1979)	5	4	24x7	100–120	10–12	48	100–200	300–500	500–1,200
26. Punia Maternity Hospital (2000)	—	1	24x7	80–90	2–3	10	100	200	500–800
27. Kajal Nursing Home (1990)	2	1	24x7	10–20	2–3	35	100	500	500–600
28. Kant Hospital (1992)	2	—	24x7	80	5–6	30	150	300	500–1,000
29. Gupta Clinic (1980)	1	—	Day	20–30	Nill	2	100	NA	NA
30. Dhir Hospital and Maternity and Eye (1992)	1	2	24x7	40–50	2	10	100	200	500–700
31. Mittal Hospital (2010)	1	—	24x7	35–40	2–3	23	100	200	500–600
32. Goel Nursing Home (1999)	1	—	24x7	30–35	1–2	10	free	200	300–500
33. Bhardwaj Maternity Hospital (1989)	3	3	24x7	50	3–5	45	100	200	500–800
34. Sangwan Hospital (2003)	1	1	24x7	18–20	1–2	7	50	100	100–250
35. Legha Bavasir Hospital (2013)	1	—	Day	10–12	Nill	4	Free	NA	NA
36. Ranvir Hospital (2008)	1	—	24x7	20–25	2–3	30	100	200	500–800
37. Sunil Dental Clinic (2003)	1	—	Day	10–15	Nill	—	30	—	—
38. Bala Ji Dental Clinic (1988)	1	1	Day	20–25	Nill	—	50	—	—
39. Narender Hospital (1982)	1	—	Day	70–80	Nill	10	50	100	300–500

Cont'd ...

... Cont'd

40.	Bohara Hospital (2004)	1	1	24x7	40–50	2–3	20	50	150	400–600
41	Ganpatrai Maternity and General Hospital (1954)	2	2	24x7	80–90	1–2	24	10	100	500–700
42	Bhardwaj Dental Hospital (2013)	1	—	Day	8–10	Nill	—	50	—	—
43	Singla Multi Speciality Hospital (2002)	4	1	24x7	40–50	3–4	28	100	300	500–800
44	GMC Hospital (2001)	2	2	24x7	60–70	4–5	35	100	200	450–950
45	Anand Nursing Home (1993)	1	—	24x7	140–150	1–2	20	150	300	100–300
46.	Ishwar Child Hospital (1997)	1	—	24x7	70–80	2–3	19	100	200	500–800
47.	Bharat Hospital (2005)	1	—	24x7	50–60	2–3	12	100	200	500–800

to obtain a random sample, therefore, non-probability or purposive sample has to be used. In this study a comprehensive sample is drawn from the universe by purposive selection method. The users of the services, i.e. the patients are selected on the basis of their length of stay in the hospital as indoor patients. The patients who minimally stayed for three days are taken into account. Since the government hospital has large number of patients, therefore, on the basis of their minimum three days stay criteria, we identified two patients daily and interviewed them for thirty days, which comes to 60 patients. In the Chug private hospital, we decided to have equal number of patients, i.e. 60 patients. Again from Chugh Private Hospital, we selected and interviewed the 60 patients on the basis of minimum of three days length of stay in the ward. Every day we interviewed 2 patients and it took 2 months to interview 60 patients from private Chugh hospital. In total, we interviewed 120 patients, 60 each from government and private hospital. We interviewed 13 doctors from government hospital and 9 doctors from private Chugh hospital. Thus, in total we interviewed 22 doctors. On the basis of several visits made to these intuitions, it became evident that there is profound difference between institutions in terms of the clinical and other facilities. Private hospitals are better equipped with latest diagnostic facilities, and good infrastructure.

IV

Data Collection

We have collected both primary and secondary data. The primary data are collected from patients and doctors from private and government hospitals. Secondary data are collected from district headquarters. We also collected information from Chief Medical Officer (CMO), State Medical Council, newspapers and journals. Data on population size, public and private health services are collected from District Census Hand Book of Bhiwani. Data are also collected from various libraries of the State and Delhi.

Interview Schedule

The elaborate interview schedule is designed to elicit the information from respondents. The schedule is always kept at hand while interviewing the respondents. A schedule is developed consisting of closed, open and multiple response questions. To confirm the responses in the schedule, the same question is asked in different ways during the interview. The responses, which are found to be consistent, are considered reliable. During all the interviews the researcher's main aim is to be completely objective and avoid any kind of bias.

Case Study

We have also taken some specific case studies of the patients pertaining to the awareness and treatment pattern, accessibility, attitudes and behaviour of the doctors. We also asked about the health rights of the patients and ethics of doctors while taking the case studies.

Focused Group Discussion

A focus group discussion is a discussion in which a small number of respondents usually between 6–12 members, under the guidance of moderator, talk about topics that are believed to be of special importance to the investigator. In recent years, there has been a notable growth in the use of focus group session research to gain insight into the dynamic relationship of attitudes, opinions, motivations, concerns and problems related to current and projected human activity. Several times, we sat outside on the ground or in the corridor of the hospital for gathering information from the patients or from their relatives and interacted with them for encountering their live experiences during the process of treatment.

V

Field Experiences

Fieldwork tradition in sociology is very common and central to sociological work. Fieldwork is the method of data collection, which provides a sociologist with first hand data based on intimate contact with the people under study. To understand the social reality of a particular society, knowledge of their environment, their history and the extent to which contact with other people has taken place is also necessary. To collect first hand information on all these aspects, sociologists engage themselves in fieldwork. Sociologists may select a particular problem for study, but try to see it with regard to its place in the total milieu and the life of the human group concerned.

Pelto and Pelto (1978) write, 'The fieldwork is the principal research instrument', the objective data collection is filtered through the subjective precautionary states of the researcher differing for various fieldworkers. Also, they differ with respect to the events and scenes that capture their interest and are aped in their predictions. Also the sociological paradigm with which a researcher identifies and views the social world of the community, apart from being conditioned by a sound theoretical knowledge, defines problems of study, methodology embraced and is again index of his/her personality and predictions. It is argued that a field situation has its unique features and it would be methodologically unsound to draw a straightjacket parallel between two fields situations. The uniqueness of any situation can be understood at two different levels. Firstly, it possesses certain challenges, in its own way to the concerned domain of sociological knowledge. Secondly, every field situation marked with its distinct physical, social, cultural and psychological milieu provides a novel situation to the fieldworker to interact with the informants. It is needless to mention here that the rules of techniques, methods and methodology are not applicable completely and it requires some flexibility in handling the field scenario. My field situation is not an exception to this. Fieldwork also involves reflexivity or critical thinking about the way one thinks. Fieldwork is thus a reflexive experience, reflecting upon one's participation.

After my registration in the Ph.D. programme, I did an extensive library work which was carried out in different libraries like Jawaharlal Nehru University, New Delhi; National Institute of Health and Family Welfare, Munrika, New Delhi; Maharshi Dayanand University, Rohtak and Punjab University, Chandigarh.

The thorough discussion with my research supervisor helped me in developing the focus of the study. After that I finalized the schedule. I was well convinced that I have to collect as much information as possible regarding medical ethics, health rights, interaction pattern of doctor-patient, etc. I was confident that I could conduct interviews, carry out observation and could establish good rapport with the patients. I collected data on socio-economic aspects of the doctors, patients, health rights and medical ethics. I also identified the various available resources, their health problems and process of seeking medical care.

The fieldwork was conducted for nearly three months in different phases. In the first phase, the study was conducted from 1 October 2013 to 30 October 2013. It is supposed to be a pilot work. The pilot study is an exploratory study that is done before beginning of the actual work. It is a pretesting of the research methods and techniques in order to perfect them. It makes one aware of difficulties beforehand and the required modifications of the techniques are made to suit field conditions. Use of a pilot can lead credence to the ability to manage qualitative research by describing initial observations on interviews.

The success of any fieldwork depends largely on the establishment of a good rapport. Rapport establishment involves the creation of a congenial atmosphere through a type of reciprocal relationship, so that the communication remains unhindered between the researcher and the respondents. A state of rapport exists between the interviewer and the informants when the latter has accepted the research goals of the interviewer and seeks to help him in obtaining the necessary information (Goode and Hatt, 1981).

As I selected two categories of respondents (i.e. patients and doctors) in government and private hospitals of Bhiwani city, I did my fieldwork in two phases. The first phase of fieldwork was conducted from 1 October 2013 to 30 October 2013, and the second phase of fieldwork from 1 November 2013 to 30 December 2013.

The first few days of fieldwork were with surveying the hospital facilities and trying to make friendship with the patients. Rapport establishment is a gradual process and often takes a long time before people come out of the 'Reactivity Syndrome' and behave in a natural way. For establishing a rapport, I tried to identify a common topic of discussion, so that there could be exchange of ideas from both sides. I slowly started involving with the patients and getting information for my interview schedule. The patients also exchanged views during conversation and narrated experiences which were quite useful for my study. In between the communication, I also explained the purpose of collecting the data for my Ph.D. work. After this phase of rapport establishment, my work was more focused, targeted and structured.

In the second phase, I started taking appointment with the doctors for getting them interviewed. Although, it is easy to tell them the purpose of taking interview but at the same time difficult to extract information. The doctors are quick in responding to the informative questions, but when the questions related to their ethical/unethical aspects of medical profession are asked, they are not quick in responding to them. Indeed, it is a tough task. Somehow, I managed to see certain situations through observation and in some situations, I verified it from the patients and other paramedical staff. However, I could collect the data and had interaction with doctors and patients, which was relevant for my research work.

Difficulties Encountered

As a researcher, I faced certain difficulties in the field. Firstly, no sociological study is available on health rights and ethics of doctors together and no secondary data is available on violation of health rights and ethics of doctors. We have general information about various cases and areas of violation of health rights in various court cases. Ethics of doctors are also not available in any systematic form.

The information, which I collected from the patients, is indeed a tough task. Patients do not want to take any risk in revealing the lapses and negligence of doctors for he/she has to again go to the doctor for his/her treatment. At another level, I faced great difficulty in collecting information from doctors because of their busy and tight schedule.

The data collected are entered in Microsoft Excel computer programme and checked for an inconsistency. The mean and percentages are calculated to compare the categorical/ dichotomized variables.

3

Health Infrastructure and Its Utilization

> Health is one of the goods of life to which man has a right; wherever this concept prevails the logical sequence is to make all measures for the protection and restoration of health to all, free of charge; medicine like education is then no longer a trade – it becomes a public function of the State.
>
> —Henry Sigerist

Health Systems have existed ever since people made systematic attempts to protect their health and treat diseases. Throughout the world, the traditional practices based on herbal cures or spiritual counselling and providing both curative and preventive care, have existed for thousands of years, and even today it has survived despite the dominance of modern medicine. The modern health system, aiming to cater to the need of a large mass of population, came into existence barely a century ago. Although in many countries, the existence of hospitals has a longer history than the organized health system. With the onset of industrial revolution, there occurred a transformation in the lives of the people, specially, in relation to health and health systems.

After World War II, interest in the word *health* resurfaced with the formation of the World Health Organization (WHO), a global entity. Around the same time, the Hygienic Laboratory in the United States was renamed the National Institutes of Health. In 1948, the World Health Organization defined health in its constitution as 'A state of complete physical, mental, and social well being and not merely the absence of disease or infirmity' (WHO, 1974). However, this definition of health has received much criticism over the years.

Medical knowledge sees health and illness as objective states that can be divorced and measured, yet this is at odds with the public perception, which is to think of health and ill health as an individual experience – as personal and unique. Our perception and understanding of the experience is shaped by the shared meanings that we possess in our culture. A disease such as cancer, for example, is often seen as an uncontrolled invasion (Sontag, 1989), and wellness is expressed through independence and control. The growing interest in the body reflects our emphasis on the individual, and it is through our bodies that we express and shape our identity. Language and visual for describing the health exists and there is a shift in the knowledge and ideas about the body so that our ways of knowing are no longer bounded by a single agreed discipline (science) but are varied and contest (cultural) (Burch, 2001).

Most of the information available on health system refers to the provision of investment in health services, i.e. health care, including curative, preventive and palliative interventions, whether directed to individuals or populations. People come into direct contact with a health system as patients attended by the health care providers. It matters very much, how the system treats people's health needs, meets their expectations, treats them with dignity, pays value to their time and anxiety, and how it raises revenues from them, including how much protection it offers them from financial risk. Again in order for an individual to utilize a service, they must believe that the service will be benefiting their health. Perceptions and motivations to use health services reveal that care is often inadequate and intensive (WHO, 1991).

Moreover, location of services and transportation problem in accessing services can be a barrier to the utilization of health facilities. Sometimes, corruption in public health services creates aversion among the care seekers. In a survey conducted in India, it was found that a quarter of all respondents had paid bribes for health services (Kumar, 2003). 'Health system includes all the activities whose primary purpose is to promote, restore or maintain health.' Real progress in health depends on strong health systems based on primary health care. Systems should integrate health promotion and disease prevention on one hand and treatment for acute illness and chronic care on the other. This should be done across all levels of health care system, with the aim of delivering quality services, equitably and efficiently to the whole population (World Health Report, 2003).

Formal health services, including professional delivery of personal medical attention, are clearly within this boundary. So are the actions by traditional healers, and all uses of medication, whether prescribed by the provider or not and the home care for sick, which is somewhere, between 70 per cent and 90 per cent of all sickness, is managed (Kleinman, 1978). At present, enhancing interventions, like roads and environment safety improvements, improvement in sanitation, educational level in general and of girls in particular – all comes under the purview of health system. The World Health Report, 2000 states that 'the health systems not only have a responsibility to improve people's health but to protect them against the financial cost of illness and to treat them with dignity'. Thus, it has identified three major objectives to develop the health systems – improving the health of the population they serve, responding to the people's expectation, and providing financial protection against the cost of ill health.

I

Health Infrastructure in India

Health is determined not only by medical care but also by determinants outside the medical sector. Public health approach is to deal with all these determinants of health which requires multi-sectoral collaboration and interdisciplinary coordination. Although there have been major improvements in public health since 1950s, India is passing through demographic and environmental transition which is adding to burden of diseases. There is triple burden of diseases, viz., communicable, non-communicable and emerging infectious diseases. This high burden of disease, disability and death can only be addressed through an effective public health system. However, the growth of public health in India has been very slow due to low public expenditure on health. Very few public health institutes in India are having adequate national standards for public health education.

Health sector in India is the responsibility of the state, local and also the central government. But in terms of service delivery it is more concerned with the state. The centre is responsible for health services in union territories without a legislature and is also responsible for developing and monitoring national standards and regulations, linking the states with funding agencies, and sponsoring numerous schemes for implementation by state governments.

The government (state, local or central) provides publicly financed and managed curative and preventive health services from primary to tertiary level, throughout the country and free of cost to the consumer. These account for about 18 per cent of the overall health spending and 0.9 per cent of the GDP. However, a fee-levying private sector that plays a dominant role in the provision of individual curative care through ambulatory services accounts for about 82 per cent of the overall health expenditure and 4.2 per cent of the gross domestic product (GDP). Goals and strategies for the public sector in health care are established through a consultative process involving all levels of government through the Central Council for Health and Family Welfare. The outcomes of these processes provide a thrust to various sub sectors within the health sector. The private and voluntary sectors have emerged as an important arm of the health sector (WHO, 2009).

Programme Implementation Division of the Government of India points out that with the exception of the states of Nagaland and Haryana, there has been 'zero per cent' growth in the setting up of primary health centres; the target was 193. The performance in terms of setting up Community Health Centres (CHC) is equally pathetic. As against the countrywide target of 103, merely 11 CHCs were set up during April 2004 and January 2005. The National Rural Health Mission (NRHM) document too draws a bleak picture – hospitalized Indians, on an average, spend 58 per cent of their total annual income on medical expenses; over 40 per cent of hospitalized Indians borrow heavily or sell their assets to cover medical expenses; over 25 per cent of hospitalized Indians fall below poverty line because of hospital expenses (GOI, 2005).

Haynes (1991) examined the relationship between socio-economic status and health services use. He found that morbidity was related to housing tenure and care availability, rather than to occupational status. He also found that age adjusted morbidity ratios were higher for females in multiple occupancy dwellings in inner city areas. Below we will discuss the different levels of health structure, in terms of Incidence of Diseases, Health Infrastructure, Pattern of Health Expenditure, and Plurality of Health Care.

Incidence or Burden of Disease

India has the highest number of Tuberculosis (TB) cases in the world. Out of 9.2 million cases of TB that occur in the world every year, nearly 1.9 million occur in India which accounts for one-fifth of the global TB cases. Experts estimate that about 2.5 million persons have HIV infection in India. This is nearly 7.6 per cent of the global burden of 33 million cases. More than 1.5 million persons are affected with malaria every year. Almost half of them suffer from falciparum malaria. One-third of global cases infected with filarial disease are in India. Nearly half of leprosy cases detected in the world in 2007 were contributed by India. More than 300 million episodes of acute diarrhoea occur every year in India in children below 5 years of age. Although data are limited, perhaps more than 35 million persons are carriers of viral hepatitis B. Emerging infectious diseases are a major public health problem in developing countries like India. Because of the existing environmental, socio-economic and demographic factors, developing countries like India are vulnerable to rapidly evolving micro-organisms. During the past three decades more than 30 new organisms have been identified worldwide including HIV, Vibrio cholera O139, SARS, corona virus, highly pathogenic avian influenza virus A, and novel H1N1 influenza virus. Many of these organisms emerged in the developing countries of Asia (Chauhan, 2011).

Globally, India accounts for half of the current leprosy cases (1.3 lakhs) and 21 per cent of Tuberculosis (TB) cases (19 lakhs). While mortality from communicable diseases has declined, there has been no decline in incidence. The new sputum positive case detection rates for Tuberculosis (TB) are less than 60 per cent in 243 districts, the Annual Parasite Index (API) for malaria continues to be above 1.9 in 142 districts, and the prevalence rate for leprosy is more than 1 per cent in 53 districts (National Institute of Health and Family Welfare, 2010).

India's achievements in the field of health leave much to be desired and the burden of disease among the Indian population remains high. Infant, children and maternal mortality and morbidity affect millions of children and women. Infectious diseases such as malaria and TB are re-emerging as epidemics and there is the growing spectre of HIV/AIDS. Many of these illness and deaths can be prevented and/or treated cost effectively with primary health care services provided by the public health system. An extensive primary health care infrastructure provided by the government exists in India. Yet, it is inadequate in terms of population coverage, especially in rural areas, and grossly underutilized because of the dismal quality of health care being provided. In most primary health care centres, drugs and equipment are missing or in short supply. There is shortage of staff and the system is characterized by endemic absenteeism on the part of medical personnel due to lack of control and oversight.

In the Indian context, the increased disease burden on the poor along with rapidly growing health care costs has been the subject of debate for some time now. Services in government health care institutions have declined over the past two decades at the primary and secondary level, leaving the sick-poor with no option but seek private health care services. Several studies have pointed out that rising expenditure on health and education is one of the main contributory factors to high indebtedness and subsequent suicides among peasants in different parts of the country in the last 10 years (Sarma, 2004).

The principal causes of infant mortality in India are prematurity, diarrhoeal diseases, acute respiratory infections, and vaccine-preventable diseases, inadequate maternal and newborn care. Malnutrition contributes to over 50 per cent of child death, low birth weight and birth injury. However, the rural-urban disparity is still a prominent determinant of receiving basic health services. India must reduce maternal mortality rate from 437 deaths per 1,00,000 live birth in 1990 to 109 by 2015. Adequate housing, water and sanitation are major issues in urban and rural development and empowerment of the poor. These issues are closely related to the quality of life, affecting multiple dimensions including psychological, sociological, cultural and economic factors (Gangadharan and Chandran, 2008).

The burden of disease also falls very unevenly on different sections of the population. The health inequalities are very sharp in India compared with many other countries including poor ones

(World Bank, 2001). Class differences in health achievements in particular are large by international standards. The same applies to gender-based inequalities in health. These features of the health situation in India relate closely to the state of health services and, going beyond that, to the persistent neglect of health matters in public policy. One symptom of this neglect is the abysmally low level of public expenditure on health – around 0.8 per cent of GDP. Among 142 countries for which the relevant data are available, only six (Burundi, Cambodia, Georgia, Indonesia, Myanmar and Sudan) have a lower figure for public expenditure on health as a proportion of Gross Domestic Product (GDP) (Dreze and Sen, 1989). The low level of public expenditure on health in India is aggravated by – a highly inefficient use of available resources, and sharp inequalities in access to health care based on region, class, caste and gender.

Health Infrastructure

Health infrastructure is an important indicator to understand the health care delivery provisions and mechanisms in a country. It also signifies the investments and priority accorded to creating the infrastructure in public and private sectors.

Health infrastructure is subdivided into two categories, viz., educational infrastructure and service infrastructure. Educational infrastructure provides details of medical colleges, students admitted to MBBS course, postgraduate degree/diploma in medical and dental colleges, admissions to BDS and MD/MS courses, AYUSH institutes, nursing courses and paramedical courses. Service infrastructure in health include details of allopathic hospitals, hospital beds, Indian System of Medicine and Homeopathy hospitals, Sub Health Centre (SHC), Primary Health Centre (PHC), Community Health Centre (CHC), blood banks, mental hospitals and cancer hospitals.

Availability of personnel and drugs often influences access to care. The nursing and paramedical staff prefers government postings. However, doctors are moving out of the public sectors. Drug availability in most public hospitals is poor; hence patients purchase medicines at the time of admission or return without care. In surgical case the list of purchases invariably includes syringes, needles, valves, lenses, etc. depending upon the nature of the surgery.

India's mandate for Universal Health Coverage (UHC) depends, to a great extent, on adequate and effective Human Resources for Health (HRH) providing care at primary, secondary and tertiary levels in both the public and private sectors. States are presently struggling with the complexities of escalating human resource costs, additional demands on the available health workforce, compounded by chronic HRH shortages, uneven distribution and skill-mix imbalances. India's health system is among the country's highest employers and absorbs almost two-thirds of the health budget for allocations in deployment, education, training, etc. Reform of HRH will, therefore, be the keystone of Universal Health Coverage reform in the country.

During the past eleven Five-Year plans, India has substantially upgraded and increased health facilities. The country presently has 1,47,069 Sub-Health Centres (SHCs), 23,673 Primary Health Centres (PHCs), 4,535 Community Health Centres (CHCs) and 12,760 hospitals in the government sector. The evidence on the actual functionality of these facilities, however, is mixed. As per the District Level Household and Facility Survey-III (DLHS, 2007–2008), 62 per cent of PHCs are conducting less than 10 deliveries in a month, 10 per cent of CHCs do not provide 24x7 normal delivery services, 34 per cent of CHCs do not have operation theatre facilities, only 19 per cent of CHCs offer caesarean section deliveries, only 9 per cent of CHCs have blood storage facilities and of the 4,535 CHCs, only 754 are functional as per IPHS (Indian Public Health Standards) norms (Ministry of Health and Family Welfare, 2011). The private health sector has grown exponentially in the country. From initially providing 8 per cent of health care facilities in 1949, the private sector now accounts for 93 per cent of the hospitals and 85 per cent of doctors in India (Khandekar, 2011).

There is an overall quantitative improvement in case of load handling. It is evident from the data that the Out-patient Department (OPD) attendance has increased from 342 million in 2006–2007 to 477 million in 2007–2008. Similarly, the indoor patient load has gone up by 155 per cent in the same time period, from 15 million to 23 million. The high focus non-North-Eastern states have shown 147 per cent increase, and the other large states have shown a 170 per cent rise. It has yet to pick up in the North-Eastern states. Jammu and Kashmir and Madhya Pradesh have shown three times the increase in OPD attendance at district hospitals. Similar improvement is evidenced in OPD attendance at the PHCs of these two states. Performance has been below par in Orissa (now Odisha) and Himachal Pradesh. Data is not available from Rajasthan and Uttar Pradesh. Among the North-Eastern states, Manipur and Tripura have shown promising improvement. It is important to note that high priority states have poorer infrastructure and much less OPD attendance to begin with, thus, after the mission, the improvement of the facilities and the scope and proportion for increase in OPD attendance could have been much more, but the result does not reflect such changes. While in large non-high focus states, where the status of utilization of services is already better, the resultant proportion of increase in

Disparities in Urban-Rural Health Facilities Distribution per Lakh Population

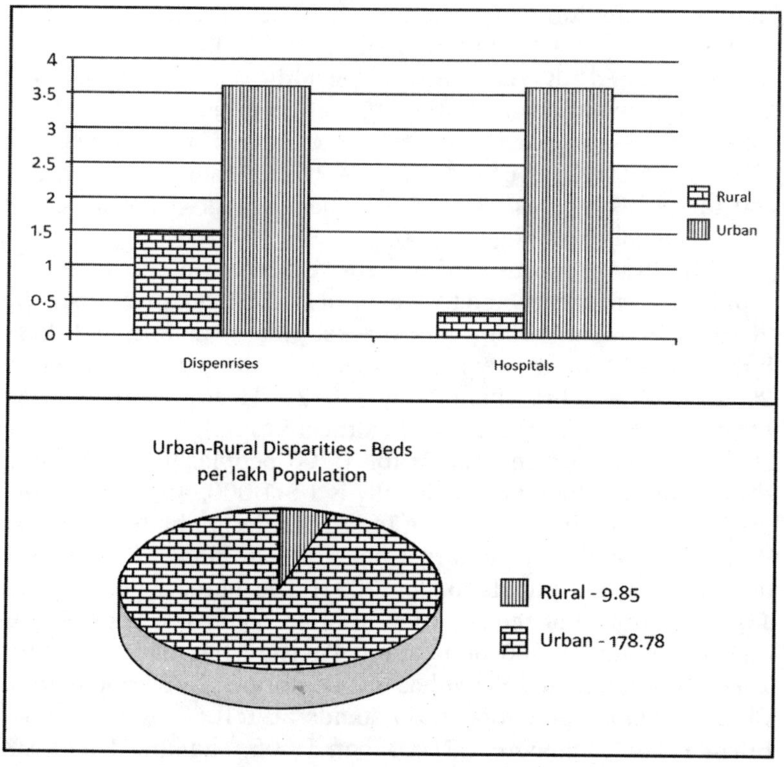

Source: Review of Health Care In India, 2005, CEHAT, Pg-S-15 to S-18, S-21.

OPD attendance is higher. This indicates a mismatch in efficient application and utilization of the mission funds in the states. However, the same is not true for the non-high focus states, except for Kerala. Nevertheless, for a majority of the non-high focus states, data is not available for 2006–2007. Wherever there has been posting of doctors and other staff and drugs have been made available, the utilization has gone up considerably (Kumar, 2011).

There are 17,000 hospitals (34% rural), 25,670 dispensaries (40% rural) and about one million beds (23% rural) at present in the country. However, the comparison between urban and rural areas shows that urban areas have 4.48 hospitals, 6.16 dispensaries and 308 beds per 1,00,000 urban population in sharp contrast to rural areas which have 0.77 hospitals, 1.37 dispensaries, 3.2 PHCs and 44 beds per 1,00,000 rural population.

Thus the urban-rural disparity is striking in spite of the fact that 70 per cent of the population comprises rural areas and only 30 per cent comprises urban areas. The shortfalls of the system are mentioned in the National Health Policy (NHP) 2002 'Applying current norms to the population projected for the year 2000, it is estimated that the shortfall in the number of SHCs/PHCs/CHCs is of the order of 16 per cent. However, this shortage is as high as 58 per cent when disaggregated for CHCs only' (Duggal and Gangolli, 2005).

The Indian health care industry is seen to be growing at a rapid pace and is expected to become a US$280 billion industry by 2020. The Indian health care market was estimated at US$35 billion in 2007 and is expected to reach over US$70 billion by 2012 and US$145 billion by 2017 (Health care.Ibef.org. http://www.ibef.org/industry/healthcare.aspx.).

India has just one doctor for 1,700 people. In comparison, the doctor population ratio globally is 1.5:1,000. An internal note prepared by Medical Council of India's 'Undergraduate Education Working Group' said the target being put in place for India is 1 doctor for 1,000 population by 2031. The note, available with TOI, also looked at the situation in other countries. Somalia has one doctor for 10,000 population, Pakistan has one doctor for 1,923 population and Egypt has one doctor per 1,484 population. China's doctor population ratio stands at 1:1063, Korea 1:951, Brazil 1:844, Singapore 1:714, Japan 1:606, Thailand 1:500, UK 1:469, US 1:350 and Germany 1:296. Currently, in India there are

330 medical colleges with an intake of approximately 35,000 students. With this intake, the shortfall of doctors by 2031 is estimated to be 9.54 lakh (*The Times of India*, 2011B).

'Planning Health Care for All' reports point out that The Planning Commission's high level expert group has given its provisional progress report on developing a framework for universal health coverage. In October 2010, Planning Commission of India with the approval of the Prime Minister, appointed a High Level Expert Group (HLEG) to develop a framework for Universal Health Coverage (UHC) to be implemented over 2010–20. The progress report has argued for universal financial protection that covers both inpatient and outpatient care under the 'evidence based belief'. Incidentally, compared to the WHO recommendation of a doctor per 1,500 population, the progress report recommends an MBBS doctor per 5,000 population. The current norm is of two MBBS doctors per Primary Health Centre (PHC) catering to 30,000 people (Phadke, 2011).

Pattern of Health Expenditure in India

The first systematic analysis of the distribution of health spending in India by source of funds, percentage of household spending, per capita spending, etc. was published in the National Health Accounts of India, 2001–02. These analyses present the pattern of health expenditure in India in detail. In this section, the distribution of public and private health expenditure and selected indicators of health expenditure is presented.

The role of the public and non-household private sector is considered to be important in reducing the burden of health care expenditure on households. It can easily be assessed that, in the absence of a well-developed non-household health care financing system, households are required to pay for the major part of health expenditure directly. The public health investments in the country over the years have been comparatively low, and as a percentage of GDP, it has declined from 1.3 per cent in 1985 to 0.8 per cent in 2002. The share of public health expenditure varies from 17 to 21 per cent in health expenditure and balance private health expenditure. Out-of-pocket payment in India is approximately 97 per cent of total private expenditure (WHO, 2003).

According to the WHO estimate, private pocket-expenditure as percentage of total health expenditure has been estimated at

80–81 per cent in India, which is much higher compared to many developing and most developed countries (WHO, 2005).

Private health care sector has grown up at a larger scale in the last few years. However private health care system is unregulated and is within reach to urban people only. It is highly affected by several factors such as technology, education and training, public expectations and perceptions, regulatory framework, societal values, etc. thus provides a high value addition to only a smaller segment. With an intention to reap profit, experience shows that the private sector is hardly concerned with public health goals, making state intervention essential. Thus, when overall health sector develops, vulnerable groups like infants, women, elderly and especially the rural segment get proportionately lesser benefit. Evidence suggests that not-for-profit sector, particularly community-based organizations, seem to have had a beneficial impact on access, equity and quality of services in rural and backward areas (Ministry of Health and Family Welfare, 2005). In such context a unique proposition in health care in the form of Public Private Partnership (PPP) was thought to be a novel strategy to bring desired result with synchronization of public goals with private sector commitments. GVK Emergency Management and Research Institute (GVK EMRI) is India's first integrated Emergency service provider operating under the PPP framework.

One major reason put forward for low level of achievement of health in India is the systematic lack of investment by the government, which adversely affects the poor. Public expenditure on health stands at less than one per cent of GDP, with state governments sharing most of the burden. In the light of economic reforms in the 1990s, the squeeze on public expenditure in health has been aggravated further especially at the state level (Mooij and Dev, 2002).

Plurality of Health Care

India has a plurality of health care systems as well as different systems of medicine. The government and local administrations provide public health care in hospitals and clinics. Public health care in rural areas is concentrated on prevention and promotion services to the detriment of curative services. The rural primary health centres are woefully underutilized because they fail to provide their clients with the desired amount of attention and medication and because they have inconvenient locations and long waiting times. Public hospitals provide 60 per cent of all hospitalizations, while the private sector provides 75 per cent of all routine care. The private sector is composed of an equal number of qualified doctors and unqualified practitioners, with a greater ratio of unqualified to qualified existing in less developed states. In rural areas, qualified doctors are clustered in areas where government services are available. With a population barely able to meet its nutritional needs, India needs universalization of health care provision to assure equity in health care access and availability instead of a large number of doctors who are profiting from the sicknesses of the poor (Duggal, 1999).

The numerous divisions of World Bank are significant forces diving privatization in health care through projects, investments and institutional support for the multinationals. The WHO also seems to be associating itself with the policy collapse into 'public-private partnership' that is taking place in other services too. These changes are being affected despite little evidence of workability and amid growing opposition from public health practitioners worldwide (Qadeer et al., 2001).

Like the public education system in India, the large public health system is also marred by endemic absenteeism and neglect on the part of health care providers. By way of incentives the employees are guaranteed a salary. There is little or no monitoring of and accountability by them. This removes any punitive pressure that acts as a corrective measure. Even the private sector, which provides most of the health services in India, is largely unregulated and there is no gate keeping on the standards of clinical practices adopted. Health care requires not only physical infrastructure and equipment, but also skilled and specialized human capital in the form of medical training and qualifications. Given the asymmetry of information between a doctor and his/her patient, low quality of medical consultancy not only lowers the efficacy of the health system but can endanger people's health. The problem of unavailability of health care personnel is two-fold, especially in rural and remote areas: (a) in many cases, rural health posts remain vacant because of unwillingness on the part of qualified doctors and other health care workers to accept placement, (b) due to lack of effective monitoring and weak or non-existent accountability, even when a post is filled, the health care provider may simply be absent. While in both cases, public health care services fail to get delivered, absenteeism is costlier because it has an associated salary burden (Chaudhury et al., 2003).

The increasing burden of diseases, insufficient infrastructure, and lower percentage of public health investment have resulted in the widening of health inequality across different sections of society. In the following section, we will discuss the health inequality.

Health Inequality

It is believed that the market system brings about efficiency and equity, and that can automatically remove all type of distortions, inadequacies and problems. However, if one examines the state of the Health Care System (HCS) in developing countries, one does not fail to observe that it is neither efficient nor equitable. These HCSs have not been able to provide markets for many types of health care goods and services; they have not been able to reduce price differences of these products within and across countries; and they have not been able to reduce inequalities in the distribution of health care goods and services (Ghosh, 2001).

India has relatively poor health outcomes, despite having a well-developed administrative system, good technical skills in many fields, and an extensive network of public health institutions for research, training and diagnosis. This suggests that the health system may be misdirecting its efforts or alternatively be poorly designed (India's Public Health System, 2004). Despite several interventions in the health care sector, the health system continues to be inadequate and insufficient to cover the population efficiently. It continues to be disconnected with public health goals, inadequately equipped to address people's expectations and fails to provide financial risk protection to those unable to access care for want of ability to pay. Accessibility and availability of a proper health care facility is still an issue. Estimated 25 per cent of people in Madhya Pradesh and Odisha could not access medical care due to reasons related to location, while it was 11 per cent for Uttar Pradesh (Ministry of Health and Family Welfare, 2005).

India adopted the Reproductive and Child Health Programme (RCHP) at the national level. Maternal health is a problem of serious proportions in India, where an estimated

1,36,000 women die needlessly each year from causes related to pregnancy, childbirth and abortion. The three countries, India, Pakistan and Bangladesh account for 28 per cent of the world's birth and 46 per cent of its maternal deaths. Maternal mortality is strongly associated with rural areas and low standards of living. For these women, access to quality health care services is difficult (Motashaw, 1997).

The strategy of identifying the poor and exempting them from user fee did not succeed. In India for example, in Andhra Pradesh green cards were supposed to be provided to the poor, but, more often than not, they went to the non-poor. In our view the strategy of depending upon Non-Governmental Organizations (NGOs) has also failed, because in most parts of India they are mainly involved in providing reproductive and child health care. In addition, their limited population coverage does not really improve access as a whole. Handing over PHC to NGOs has also not worked in India due to political and administrative constraints.

The issue of inequality of health care services is a serious matter in less developed countries. There are indeed many types of inequalities in the distribution of medical care services in these countries. For instance, doctor-population ratio, numbers of hospitals and medical clinics per unit of population vary substantially from region to region. It is one of the duties of the government to make the distribution pattern more and more egalitarian as far as possible, so that inequalities in many health indicators across the country such as the infant mortality rate and life expectancy can be eradicated in the long run. Good health is so fundamental to human life and existence that it cannot be left to the dictates of market forces. In fact, health has come to be regarded as a more fundamental responsibility of the government than even education, and hence health deserves more egalitarianism and equity considerations (Stiglitz, 1998).

After discussing the health inequality across different sections of society, we will trace back the development of health care and different health polices over a period of time.

Health Care Development and Health Policy

Health is regarded as an important form of human capital formation and benefits of improving health status are far reaching.

The health status of a population measures the quality of life of the people. It is both an end in itself and a means to achieve other ends. There are compelling arguments for accelerating investment in health. Good health is considered to be an integral part of development. Further, it contributes to increasing the productivity of the economically active population which in turn enhances earnings. Health also accounts for longevity and well-being of children and the aged population. The benefit of good health both to the individual in whom it is embodied as well as to the society at large are so pervasive that health investments is accorded high priority everywhere (Sen, 1999).

Health care is one of the key parameters in which a country's development and status are measured. The provision of health under Indian constitution falls in State list. Today, every state is free to formulate their health programme and strategy. In fact, India was the first country in the world, which introduced family planning programme in 1952. The government provides a three-tier (Primary, Secondary and Tertiary) support structure for addressing the health care needs across the country.

Over the last 50 years, India has achieved a lot in terms of health improvement. But still, India is way behind many fast developing countries such as China, Vietnam and Sri Lanka in terms of health indicators. In case of government funded health care system, the quality and access of services has always remained a major concern. A very rapidly growing private health market has developed in India. This private sector bridges most of the gaps between what government offers and what people need (Satia et al., 1999).

Two areas critical to a robust and efficient medical care system are emergency and specialist medical care. Emergency care is still in a very nascent stage all across India, while specialist medical care is markedly better for the urban, middle-and upper-class Indians than for their less wealthy counterparts (both rural and urban). The current Emergency Medical Services (EMS) infrastructure is inefficient due to the lack of critical components such as: a centralized administrative body, trained emergency medical personnel, a centralized emergency phone number (similar to '911'), and quality ambulance services. There are, however, signs of change in EMS due to an increase in the number of government initiatives.

The quality and availability of specialist medical care varies greatly among the different socio-economic groups and by geography, i.e. urban vs. rural. Despite a high annual output of medical specialist graduates, specialist medical care has traditionally been very poor in India due to 'brain drain', or the phenomena of highly educated Indians immigrating to western countries. Recently, however, specialist care for the middle- and upper-classes has improved due to more private hospitals, better private hospital infrastructures and equipment, and higher salaries/incentives (mostly a result of increased demand from the growing middle-class).

The relevance of this issue of equity is further highlighted by the fact that despite higher utilization of the private sector on the whole, in case of serious illness a greater proportion of the poor seek public hospitals. It is also known that ill health is a major cause of indebtedness and economic pressure in rural areas. Inevitably, pushing privatization of medical care in regions where both the degree and proportion of service deprivation are high, transforms privatized health care into a tool for marginalization (Iyer and Sen, 2000).

As a result, most people in India, even the poor, choose expensive health care services provided by the largely unregulated private sector. Not only do the poor face the double burden of poverty and ill health, but also the financial burden of ill health can push even the non-poor into poverty. On the other hand, a healthy population is instrumental for poverty reductions and economic growth, two important developmental goals. In India, public spending on health is less than 1 per cent of its GDP, which is grossly inadequate. Public investment in health, particularly in primary health care needs to be much higher to achieve health targets, to reduce poverty and to raise the rate of economic growth. Moreover, the health system needs to be reformed to ensure efficient and effective delivery of good quality health services (Bajpai, 2010).

More than thirty-six years after the 'Health for All' declaration was signed, evidence suggests that improving the health of the poorest group in India remains an immense challenge. Researchers tend to agree that the most effective response to health disparities are multi-sector, involving health, education, labour and other sectors. The approaches for improving the health status of the poor can be broadly classified as socio-economic approaches, health services approaches and health financing approach (Evans, 2001).

To track progress towards achieving the goal related to maternal, newborn and child survival, a movement named 'Countdown to 2015' was initiated by various stakeholders including governments, individuals and institutions. The countdown is aimed to stimulate country-specific action by tracking coverage, health system performance measures and policies and interventions needed to achieve these Millennium Development Goals (MDGs). It places India among a set of 68 countries having the highest burden of maternal and child mortality (UNICEF, 2008).

To mention the development in health, we need to have health policies. The health policies are prioritized on the basis of planning. The aim of health policy is to secure a fundamental change in health status of people. Health policies also include the decisions on medical education, health facilities, health coverage, medical research, choice of systems of medicine, etc. It also includes the decisions as regards the relative role of the government, the private and voluntary agencies in the promotion of health care. The health policy must be made with relevance to the time dimension. It can be a long-term policy. In both developed and developing countries governments have been centrally involved in health regulation and provision, ranging from public health measures that ensure safe water and unadulterated food, to border controls that attempts to regulate the spread of communicable diseases.

Health care planning in India has a number of objectives. Among the three important objectives are (a) keeping up with modern development in the field of all allopathic and other medicines, (b) making medical care and medical education relevant to India's needs, and (c) increasing the access of the masses to the modern and other medicines. Several committees appointed by the central government since Independence have periodically reviewed the progress made in health planning. Alternative viewpoints for a health policy are also relevant to the conditions and provide a wider access to health care to its people. Various aspects of the National Health Policy of India 2002 along with recent National Rural Health Mission of 2005 have also been examined in this chapter.

Health Policy for all by the Year 2000 AD

The access to the basic health care facilities is a common phenomenon in most of the developing countries. In order to provide minimum basic health facilities, it was resolved by the Health Assembly of the WHO to launch a movement known as 'Health for All by the Year 2000 AD'. In 1978, the Alma-Ata conference reaffirmed Health for All as the major social goal of all governments. In 1981, a global strategy for this programme was adopted by the WHO, which was later endorsed by the United Nations General Assembly. India is a signatory to those declarations and has made efforts to extend health facilities to the vulnerable sections of its society. Health for All has been defined as attainment of 'a level of health that will enable every individual to lead a socially and economically productive life' (Government of India, 1983).

The concept of 'Health for All by the Year 2000 AD' implied a substantial change in basic health policies and in the approaches to health care. In order to provide minimum health facilities, the government of India along with state governments increased the allocation to the health sector. On the whole, it appeared that there was tremendous investment in widening the health infrastructure, which included within its purview a variety of programmes and viewed health and humans as a vital component of overall socio-economic development.

A group set up jointly by the ICSSR and ICMR with Dr Ramalingaswami as the Chairman came up with an alternative strategy to achieve health for all citizens. It suggested certain steps for restructuring the health care service infrastructure based on the principle of promoting the preventive and curative aspects of health. This group felt that, 'the growth of health care services in the country has been haphazard and unrelated to the needs of poor and rural people who stand most in need of health care'. The group remarked that several assumptions on which present system is based were wrong. For instance, there was no distinction between planning for *health* and that for *health services* so that little or no attention has been paid to the social, economic, political and cultural dimensions of health. The recommendations of the study group were more practical and provided details of health services up to the village level. It emphasized that most common illness can be self-cured and need only symptomatic treatment with simple remedies, be it herbal, indigenous or allopathic medicine. The diseases, which are communicable, can be controlled by preventive measures, and can be readily diagnosed and treated with the help of cheap and highly effective drugs. The group, therefore, proposed that primary health services should be extended to the community through a trained and involved community health volunteer preferably male or female, for a population of 1,000. The study group has recommended the elimination of the PHC category as it feels that it is an institution of semi-professional and paramedical personnel who deliver poor medical care and extend no preventive promotive health care (ICSSR and ICMR, 1981). To lift the status of preventive and promotive aspects of medical services, the working group has suggested that greater emphasis be given to departments of preventive and social medicine, which are currently underdeveloped. By improving the status of women, we can hope to give better quality health to the population. Thus, the group provides details on the services and their components needed for improving the health of the people such as education, environmental conditions, level of nutrition and employment.

Health Policy, 1983

The historical development reflected through various Plan Documents and Policy Directions (1982) brings out explicit actions on inter-sectoral cooperation not only of different developmental sectors but also of various intra-sectoral efforts in the field of health, family planning, education and research, drugs, pharmaceuticals, agriculture, food, water supply and drainage, housing, education, social welfare, rural development, etc.

NHP-1983 health policy, develops a rationale for a new health policy, defines a framework for health sector reforms, argues for structural changes within the context of a universal health care approach and evolves the framework. Several pertinent issues in health sector reforms have a bearing on our constitutional provisions like: equity, accessibility of poor, efficiency in using resources and inadequacy of resources, gender bias, quality of health care, impact of liberalization, etc. The changed circumstances relating to the health sector of the country since 1983 generated a situation in which National Health Policy-2002 has been formulated.

National Health Policy, 2002

The main objective of this policy is to achieve an acceptable standard of good health amongst the general population of the country. The approach would be to increase access to the decentralized public health system by establishing new infrastructure in deficient areas, and by upgrading the infrastructure in the existing institutions. Overriding importance would be given to ensuring a more equitable access to health services across the social and geographical expanse of the country. Emphasis will be given to increasing the aggregate public health investment through a substantially increased contribution by the Central Government. It is expected that this initiative will strengthen the capacity of the public health administration at the State level to render effective service delivery. The contribution of the private sector in providing health services would be much enhanced, particularly for the population group, which can afford to pay for services. Primacy is given to preventive and first-line curative initiatives at the primary health level through increased sectoral share of allocation. Emphasis is be laid on rational use of drugs within the allopathic system. Increased access to tried and tested system of traditional medicine is also ensured.

The public health investment in the country over the years has been completely low, and as percentage of GDP has declined from 1.3 per cent in 1990 to 0.9 per cent in 1999. The aggregate expenditure in the health sector is 5.2 per cent of the GDP. Out of this, about 17 per cent of the aggregate expenditure is on public health spending, the balance being out-of-pocket expenditure. The central budgetary allocation for health over this period, as a percentage of the total central budget, has been stagnant at 1.3 per cent, while that in the states declined from 7.0 per cent to 5.5 per cent. The current annual per capita public health expenditure in the country was not more than ₹ 200 (Government of India, 2002).

In the period when centralized planning was accepted as a key instrument of development in the country, the attainment of an equitable regional distribution was considered one of its major objectives. Despite this conscious focus in the development process, the attainment of health indices has been very uneven across the rural-urban divide, e.g. infant mortality in rural area was 75 per thousand, whereas in urban area it is 44 per thousand (Government of India, 2002).

To meet the objective of reducing various types of inequalities and imbalances inter regional, across the rural-urban divide, and between economic classes the most cost-effective method would be to increase the sectoral outlay in the primary health sector. Such outlets afford access to a vast number of individuals, and also facilitate preventive and early stage curative initiative, which were cost effective. In recognition of this public health principle, NHP-2002 sets out an increased allocation of 55 per cent of the total public health investment for the primary health sector, the secondary and tertiary health sector being targeted for 35 per cent and 10 per cent respectively. The policy projects that the increased aggregate outlays for the primary health sector will be utilized for strengthening existing facilities and opening additional public health service outlets, consistent with the norm for such facilities.

In principle, this policy welcomes the participation of the private sector in all areas of health activities – primary, secondary or tertiary. The policy also encourages the setting up of private insurance instruments for increasing the scope of the coverage of the secondary and tertiary sector under private health insurance packages. Under the overreaching umbrella of the national heath framework, the alternative systems of medicine – Ayurveda, Unani, Siddha and Homeopathy – have a substantial role. Because of inherent advantages, such as diversity, modest cost, low level of technological input and the growing popularity of natural plant-based products, these systems are attractive, particularly in the underserved, remote and tribal areas. The alternative systems will draw upon the substantial untapped potential of India as one of the eight important global centres for plant diversity in medicinal and aromatic plants.

National Rural Health Mission (NRHM), 2005

NRHM was launched on 12 April 2005 in 18 states to provide comprehensive integrated health care to rural people, especially vulnerable sections of the society – women and children. One of the key components of the project was to provide every village with trained female community health activist, known as ASHA (Accredited Social Health Activist). She would be selected from the village itself and be accountable to the panchayat. She would be the interface between the community and the public health system. These ASHAs get no remuneration, were provided only performance-incentives for reproductive and child health and other programmes. They get an average of ₹ 1,100 a month this way and were equipped with drug-kit containing drugs for common ailments.

Union Health Secretary, P.K. Hota, has stated, 'It is a massive project aimed at providing basic health care to villagers. Though the centre has framed all the policy and extended all support for the project, it is the state government who has to implement it. For NRHS, for 2006–2007 the health ministry earmarked ₹ 120 crore and which has almost been spent. But even 10 months after the launch of the ambitious ₹ 6,714 crore NRHM project it has hardly taken off. Even recruitment of 2.5 lakh voluntary female health workers as per the schemes has not reached the half way (*The Times of India*, 2006).

Drug Policy

Drug policy is related to the drug industry. The first comprehensive drug policy of 1978 has been scrapped by the government. The number of drugs targeted under price control declined from 343 to 73 in 1994. The profitability allowed in these categories also increased, from 40 to 75 per cent in 1987 to 150 per cent in 1994. Even this scale of profits is to be rendered redundant soon, as the drugs under control are to be further reduced (FMRAI, 2001).

A drug committee identifies the list of essential drugs. It consists of professors of medicine, clinicians in various medical fields, pharmacologists, a representative from the World Health Organization, health secretary and the managing director of Tamil Nadu Medical Services Corporation (TNMSC). All government health care institutions and pharmacists are given the list of essential drugs. Thereafter, local health officials can request the committee to modify the list in accordance with their local needs. The drugs allocated to PHCs are limited to 54 essential drugs. TNMSC invites tenders by advertising in the print media, including pharmaceutical trade journals and its own website, with clear guidelines for supplier selection, quality control and distribution. The committee pays the supplier only after receiving a report on quality control. A detailed system of warehousing the drugs and accounting by the health centre are a part of the procurement policy (Lalitha, 2007).

Health policy in India, like all public policy, has always been the product of complex political processes. In the area of women's health, the situation is further complicated by the fact that policy processes have to straddle a treacherous faultline between target-driven population-control goals on the one hand, and issues of individual reproductive rights and general well-being on the other (Pachauri, 1994).

India, over the last two decades, has enjoyed accelerated economic growth, but has fared poorly in human development indicators and health outcomes. Population averages of health status indicators, such as child health and maternal mortality, remain unacceptably high compared with countries in the South and East Asian regions that have similar income levels and rates of economic growth. Underlying the low population level indicators, worrisome inequities coincide with the multiple axes of caste, class, gender and regional differences (Deaton and Dreze, 2009).

The private sector, constituting both 'for profit' and 'non-profit' institutions, has a sizeable presence in delivery of health services, which comprises a wide array of institutions with varying degrees of sophistication in terms of services and qualified personnel. The 'for profit' sector is proportionately larger than the 'non-profit' sector; the latter includes community level programmes, dispensaries and hospitals that are funded by religious and secular organizations (Nundy, 2005).

Nagla (1993) has highlighted the enormous efforts made by the various committees to chart out the growth of health manpower in India. The works of these committees have, been subject to serious data limitations. Information on different categories of health personnel, their priorities and distribution (especially in respect to professionals outside the public sector) has been rather scanty. The various committees and even institutions like the ICSSR/ICMR study groups have been focusing on providing expert opinion rather than garnering accurate statistical data. No committee has been able to take into account the contribution of non-governmental health institutions and that of professionals in rendering health care services. After discussing the health care development and health polices over a period of time, now we turn below to discuss health infrastructure in our area of study, i.e. Haryana.

II

Health Infrastructure in Haryana

In Haryana, the health situation of its people is also not very impressive. It accounts for 11.1 per cent child mortality rate, 22 per cent crude birth rate, 72.3 per cent anaemic children, 27 per cent malnutrition among women, 56.1 per cent anaemic women and 41.7 per cent infant mortality rate. Even 72.3 per cent households do not generally use government health facilities due to poor quality of care (NFHS, 2005–06).

Table 3.1 shows the health infrastructure in Haryana.

Table 3.1

Health Infrastructure of Haryana

Health Infrastructure	*Required*	*In position*	*Shortfall*
Sub-centre	4,159	2,520	1,639
Primary Health Centre	657	447	210
Community Health Centre	164	109	55
Health worker (Female)/ANM at Sub Centres and PHCs	2,967	4,973	—
Health Worker (Male) at Sub Centres	2,520	1,682	838
Health Assistant (Female)/LHV at PHCs	447	398	49
Health Assistant (Male) at PHCs	447	503	—
Doctor at PHCs	447	342	105
Obstetricians and Gynaecologists at CHCs	109	11	98
Pediatricians at CHCs	109	10	99
Total specialists at CHCs	436	29	407
Radiographers at CHCs	109	142	—
Pharmacist at PHCs and CHCs	556	880	—
Laboratory Technicians at PHCs and CHCs	556	394	162
Nurse/Midwife at PHCs and CHCs	1,210	1,698	—

Source: RHS Bulletin, March 2012, M/O Health and F.W., GOI.

The state of Haryana is trying to achieve the good health care for all by the year of 2012. The number of hospitals, dispensaries and health centre as 3,073 followed by 474 Ayurvedic, Unani and Homeopathic institutions with the facility of the family welfare centres where 10,944 beds are available and 86.38 lakh patient are treated. These medical facilities are available at either the headquarters of the district, tehsil and block or at the urban centres to facilitate the medical services to 6,678 villages and 106 towns (Ansari, 2005).

Health Policy in Haryana

Haryana's former Chief Minister Om Prakash Chautala, on 27 October 2003, announced that all senior citizens over 60 years of age would be provided health services free of cost. The chief minister, who made this announcement while inaugurating a health camp at Idri village in Nuh subdivision, said that a dentist would also be appointed at each health centre in the state. The state government has also decided to provide 225 medicines free of cost to patients, revealed Chautala, claiming that Haryana was the first state in the country to do this. He also directed the health authorities that those patients who were seriously sick and diagnosed at this camp be provided free medical aid in Delhi and at other places also (*The Times of India*, 2003).

With growing population and industrialization, health care services are still way below standards in Haryana, obviously on account of lack of adequate infrastructure, coupled with shortage of doctors and other medical staff. According to health department figures, there are 111 CHCs, 332 PHCs and 2,603 sub-health centres in the state, leaving a wide gap in terms of population-health care institution ratio of the Central Government. Dr Kuldeep Singh, a medical officer and president of Haryana Civil Medical Services Association, Rohtak, maintained that with around 2.14 crore population, there is a need for 165 CHCs, 551 PHCs and 3,306 sub-centres in Haryana. Talking to TOI (*The Times of India*), he said that as per public health standards set by Union Ministry of Health and Family Welfare, there should be one sub-centre per 5,000 people, one PHC per 30,000 people and one CHC per one lakh population. In Haryana, over 75 per cent live in rural areas and it was not possible for majority of people to access qualified and costly medical care even in urban areas (*The Times of India*, 2011A).

The problem does not end here as available health care centres are grappling with shortage of doctors. There are around 600 posts lying vacant, even though the department had been trying to fill the vacancies, but medical officers were quitting obviously due to lack of job incentives. Even in Rohtak district, which is home district of Haryana chief minister Bhupinder Singh

Hooda, 34 posts of medical officers are lying vacant in CHCs and PHCs. The Haryana Civil Medical Services Association (HCMSA) president said that doctors have been quitting due to comparatively low salary package in comparison to Punjab, Himachal, Rajasthan, Uttar Pradesh and Delhi, apart from poor career incentive policies.

Existing Health Centres	*Required Number as per Population*	
(i) Sub-centres	2,603	3,306
(ii) PHCs	332	551
(iii) CHCs	111	165

Source : The Times of India: 11 November 2011A.

In the ensuing chapters, we will analyse the data collection from the field situation in terms of conception of health, health rights of patients and ethics of doctors.

4

Socio-Economic Background of Patients and Doctors

The expectations of patients differ according to their life circumstances and basic personality disposition. When a patient enters the hospital, he brings with him a set of beliefs, attitudes, values and social relationships. The socio-economic background of the patient, his cultural attitudes, education, values and earlier experiences of self as well as those of his relatives are important determinants of how he will react to hospitalization and the services rendered by various personnel in the hospital. In the modern society, educational status has become very important in determining one's socio-economic conditions; education brings a kind of awareness towards the existing social set-up and a consciousness about the existing facilities in the society. Education plays a role towards bringing changes in the society. It forms a social group based on achievement that represents a social class.

In every social system, the interaction and interrelationship between its members in accordance with the goals and the institutional sanctions is the basis for the functioning of the system. The hospital is considered here as a social system and the doctors and patients are the sole occupants who mutually interact to form relationship directed by their specific goals and the general goals of the system. The entire organization and instrumentality within this system has its concern with the social aspects of human behaviour. Thus, the forms, patterns and directions of the relationship with their bearing on the goals and norms of this collectivity have to be ascertained in relation to the functioning of the system with reference to the doctors, patients and their satisfaction in a given situation, existing in a hospital at a particular time.

The patients have to depend entirely on medical professionals for their recovery. The risk of the patient's life forces him to do as the doctors say. This, therefore, becomes a necessity that the doctors possess high moral character and maintain high professional ethics. If the societal system gives way for the fulfilment of individual self-interests of the professionals the patients are likely to suffer more. The poor patients, who do not have any means of support, suffer most in this process.

In the proceeding pages, we will discuss the socio-economic background of patients and doctors. The chapter is divided into two sections. In the first section we will discuss the socio-economic profile of patients and in Section two we will dwell upon doctors' socio-economic background.

I

Socio-Economic Background of Patients

Health behaviour is strongly determined by the different social, economic, education and environmental circumstances of individuals and populations. Improvement of health literacy can help individuals to tackle the determinants of health better as it builds up the personal, cognitive and social skills which determine the ability of individuals to gain access to, understand and use information to promote and maintain good health.

Table 4.1

Nativity of Patients

Nativity	*Government Hospital*	*Private Hospital*	*Total*
Rural	38 (31.67)	40 (33.33)	78 (65)
Urban	22 (18.33)	20 (16.67)	42 (35)
Total	60 (50)	60 (50)	120 (100)

Figures in the bracket represent percentage.

Table 4.1 shows that 78 (65%) patients are from rural area who are seeking treatment in government and private hospital, whereas only 35 per cent belong to urban area. It clearly shows that India is a country of villages. Urban areas are having a mushrooming growth of private health care and at the same time there is an absence of government health care facilities in rural areas, forcing people to the urban areas for seeking treatment.

Table 4.2

Age-Group of the Patients

Age (in Years)	*Government Hospital*	*Private Hospital*	*Total*
1–20	13 (10.83)	2 (1.67)	15 (12.5)
21–30	12 (10)	20 (16.67)	32 (26.67)
31–40	13 (10.83)	8 (6.667)	21 (17.5)
41–50	9 (7.5)	10 (8.33)	19 (15.83)
51–60	6 (5)	5 (4.17)	11 (9.17)
61–70	5 (4.17)	10 (8.33)	15 (12.5)
71 and above	2 (1.67)	5 (4.17)	7 (5.83)
Total	60 (50)	60 (50)	120 (100)

Figures in the bracket represent percentage.

Table 4.2 shows that there are only 2 (1.67%) patients from age-group of 1–20 years. There are 20 (16.67%) patients from age-group of 21–30 in private hospital. Again, there are only 2 (1.67%) patients who are above 70 years of age in government hospital.

Table 4.3

Caste and Gender Category of Patients

Caste/Category	*Government Hospital*		*Private Hospital*		*Total*
	Male	*Female*	*Male*	*Female*	
General*	12 (10)	4 (3.37)	9 (7.5)	10 (8.33)	35 (29.16)
OBC**	16 (13.33)	9 (7.5)	18 (15)	20 (16.67)	63 (52.5)
SC***	14 (11.67)	5 (4.16)	3 (2.5)	—	22 (18.33)
Total	42 (35)	18 (15)	30 (25)	30 (25)	120 (100)

Figures in the bracket represent percentage.

* General Category includes: Brahmin, Baniya, Khatri, Arora.

**Other Backward Caste includes: Jat, Yadav, Mali, Khati, Nai, Kumhar.

*** Scheduled Caste includes: Dhanak, Chamar, Valmiki.

Table 4.3 shows that out of 29.16 per cent of general category patients, there are 10 per cent male patients in government hospital. Nearly seventeen per cent female patients in OBC category are taking treatment from private hospital. There are total of 52.5 per cent patients in government and private hospital from OBC category which is the highest among all the three categories. Thus, there is a preponderance of patients from other backward caste.

Table 4.4

Marital Status of the Patients

Marital Status	*Government Hospital*	*Private Hospital*	*Total*
Married	39 (32.5)	42 (35)	81 (67.50)
Unmarried	17 (14.17)	9 (7.5)	26 (21.67)
Widow	4 (3.33)	9 (7.5)	13 (10.83)
Total	60 (50)	60 (50)	120 (100)

Figures in the bracket represent percentage.

Table 4.4 shows that there is majority of married patients in government and private hospital which is 67.50 per cent of total patients. There are 14.17 per cent unmarried patients in government hospital. Most of the patients who are widows are in private hospital which is 7.5 per cent of total 10.83 per cent widow patients.

Table 4.5

Income-Group of the Patients

Annual Income-Group (in ₹)	*Government Hospital*	*Private Hospital*	*Total*
Less than fifty thousand	10 (8.33)	1 (.83)	11 (9.17)
More than fifty thousand to one lakh	31 (25.83)	18 (15)	49 (40.83)
More than one lakh to three lakh	17 (14.17)	33 (27.5)	50 (41.67)
More than three lakh to five lakh	2 (1.67)	6 (5)	8 (6.67)
More than five lakh and above	—	2 (1.67)	2 (1.67)
Total	60 (50)	60 (50)	120 (100)

Figures in the bracket represent percentage.

Table 4.5 shows that majority of the patients, i.e. 50 (41.67%) are having their income more than one lakh to three lakh and within that there are 33 (27.5%) patients from the same income group who are taking treatment from private hospital. There is only 1 (0.83%) patient who is having income below fifty thousand rupees. There are no patients in government hospital who are having their income above five lakh.

Table 4.6

Gender and Income-Group of Patients

Annual Income (in ₹)	*Government Hospital*		*Private Hospital*		*Total*
	Male	*Female*	*Male*	*Female*	
Less than fifty thousand	7 (5.83)	3 (2.5)	1 (.83)	—	11 (9.17)
More than fifty thousand to one lakh	23 (19.17)	8 (6.67)	11 (9.17)	7 (5.83)	49 (40.83)
More than one lakh to three lakh	11 (9.17)	6 (5)	16 (13.33)	17 (14.17)	50 (41.67)
More than three lakh to five lakh	1 (.83)	1 (.83)	1 (.83)	5 (4.17)	8 (6.67)
More than five lakh and above	—	—	1 (.83)	1 (.83)	2 (1.67)
Total	42 (35)	18 (15)	30 (25)	30 (25)	120 (100)

Figures in the bracket represent percentage.

Table 4.6 shows that there is no female patient in the private hospital whose income is less than fifty thousand. This shows that female patients are having less income. Table also indicates that high profile income group prefers the private hospital for treatment instead of government hospital. Out of total, 40.83 per cent male and female patients who are having income more than fifty thousand to one lakh income, are taking treatment in government hospital which is highest among the entire income group. Little more than 40 per cent patients are having income between one lakh to three lakh.

There are special/private wards within the government and private hospitals; therefore we have tried to understand the frequency of patients in special/private ward. Table 4.7 shows that 10 (8.33%) patients from less than fifty thousand income group are in general ward of government hospital. It shows that people think that if they want to avail the private ward facility within the government hospital, it is better to go in the private hospital, where they can also have easy access to the doctor and much better facilities. In private hospital, there is a trend that the higher the income group, the more patient opt for special ward. All patients from five lakh and above income group are taking treatment in special ward of private hospital (see Table 4.7).

Table 4.7

Income-Group and Ward of Patients

Annual Income (in ₹)	*Government Hospital*		*Private Hospital*		*Total*
	General ward	*Private ward*	*General ward*	*Private/ Special ward*	
Less than fifty thousand	10 (8.33)	—	—	1 (.83)	11 (9.17)
More than fifty thousand to one lakh	29 (24.17)	2 (1.67)	15 (12.5)	3 (2.5)	49 (40.83)
More than one lakh to three lakh	16 (13.33)	1 (0.83)	13 (10.83)	20 (16.67)	50 (41.67)
More than three lakh to five lakh	—	2 (1.67)	1 (0.83)	5 (4.17)	8 (6.67)
Five lakh and above	—	—	—	2 (1.67)	2 (1.67)
Total	55 (45.83)	5 (4.17)	29 (24.17)	31 (25.83)	120 (100)

Figures in the bracket represent percentage.

Table 4.8

Patients and their Type of Family

Type of Family	*Government Hospital*	*Private Hospital*	*Total*
Joint	33 (27.5)	25 (20.83)	58 (48.33)
Nuclear	27 (22.5)	35 (29.17)	62 (51.67)
Total	60 (50)	60 (50)	120 (100)

Figures in the bracket represent percentage.

Table 4.8 represents that most of the patients 62 (51.67%), belong to nuclear family and out of that 35 (29.17%)

patients are taking treatment from the private hospital. In the government hospital there are 33 (27.5%) patients who belong to joint family. Thus, we can conclude that people from Joint family prefer to take treatment in government hospital as they have more number of members in their household who can better look after their patients.

Table 4.9 shows that one-fifth of patients, i.e. 20 (16.67%) patients who are taking treatment in government hospital are illiterate. It clearly shows that illiterate patients are coming to government hospital as they do not have purchasing power of buying the health care. And 16 (13.33%) patients who are taking treatment in private hospital are graduates. The table shows that higher educated patients go to private hospital instead of government hospital to take treatment. There are no patients who are graduate and taking treatment in government hospital.

Table 4.9

Educational Level of Patients

Level of Education	*Government Hospital*	*Private Hospital*	*Total*
Illiterate	20 (16.67)	18 (15)	38 (31.67)
Primary	9 (7.5)	6 (5)	15 (12.5)
Middle	14 (11.67)	5 (4.17)	19 (15.83)
Matriculation	6 (5)	4 (3.33)	10 (8.33)
10+2	8 (6.67)	7 (5.83)	15 (12.5)
BA/BEd	3 (2.5)	16 (13.33)	19 (15.83)
MA/MSc	—	4 (3.33)	4 (3.33)
Total	60 (50)	60 (50)	120 (100)

Figures in the bracket represent percentage.

Table 4.10 indicates that there are 18 (15%) patients in government hospital whose occupation is agricultural labour/farmer and 10 (8.33%) patients, who have clerical job or skilled work, go to the private hospital. However, there are no patients of teaching and other professions who are seeking treatment in government hospital. There are 19 (15.83%) unemployed/students/old-aged patients who are taking treatment from government hospital.

Table 4.10
Occupation of Patients

Type of Occupation	*Patients in Government Hospital*	*Patients in Private Hospital*	*Total*
House wives	11 (9.17)	14 (11.67)	25 (20.83)
Agricultural labour/construction labour/farmer	18 (15)	6 (5)	24 (20)
Petty shopkeeper or small business	5 (4.17)	6 (5)	11 (9.17)
Clerical job/skilled work	6 (5)	10 (8.33)	16 (13.33)
Teaching and other professions	—	4 (3.33)	4 (3.33)
Unemployed/old age/students	19 (15.83)	14 (11.67)	33 (27.5)
Ex-servicemen	1 (.83)	6 (5)	7 (5.83)
Total	60 (50)	60 (50)	120 (100)

Figures in the bracket represent percentage.

II

Socio-Economic Background of Doctors

Profession of medicine has grown and developed within the societal framework of our country (Nagla, 1997). The doctors who are involved in the task of general practice, after all, belong to some ethnic group; they have a social background of caste and class, they belong to some religious sects and what is more, they are ideologically oriented to the realms of voluntary services. They are in fact products of the prevailing education system, along with both its merits and demerits. They have a family life, a spouse and children. His performance as general practitioner is thus determined by his social conditioning including his economic status. Yet another important factor which conditions the professionals in medicine are the working conditions of the hospital system. Whether a doctor is employed in government run hospitals, charitable hospitals, public health centres, dispensaries or privately run clinics, they want some system of reward. They wish to get some satisfaction out of the job they are doing. They would also aspire for accumulation of money. There are a number of inducements and incentives which enable them to do their job successfully. When we argue that the practitioners do not get satisfaction from the available working conditions, namely, salary scale, remuneration, opportunities of promotion facilities for the upbringing of family, the outcome of their practice would not be satisfactory. The medical profession, therefore, has multidimensions. It is inclusive of the social background of the medical practitioners, the processes of admission to medical education, training and acquisition of skills, working conditions and above all, importantly enough, the ethics of the profession. In the present chapter we would make an attempt to dwell on socio-economic background of doctors with strength of data generated by us from the field.

Doctors and their Gender Category

Out of the total sample, there are 12 male and 10 female doctors who are serving in private and government hospital (Table 4.11). It is a clear indication that now female doctors' ratio is increasing in the medical profession also. Earlier there was a low representation of females in all professions including medical profession. It is also found in some empirical studies on medical profession in India that there is a low ratio of female professionals as compared to male (Madan, 1980; Venkatratnam, 1979). Most women doctors prefer gynaecology, paediatrics, obstetrics, anaesthesia and pathology. Madan (1972, 1980) also found in his study that 'in actual practice, all of the lady doctors function as specialists concentrating on the treatment of women and children'.

Table 4.11

Gender Category of Doctors

Gender Category	*Government Hospital*	*Private Hospital*	*Total*
Male	7 (31.82)	5 (22.73)	12 (54.54)
Female	6 (27.28)	4 (18.18)	10 (45.46)
Total	13 (59.09)	9 (40.91)	22 (100)

Figures in the bracket represent percentage.

Age-Group of Doctors

The age-group of doctor's range from 25–51 years and above. We find that those holding senior positions among doctors are mostly in the age-group of 36–51 years. The preponderance of doctors in the age-group of 25–35 years, while they obtain the MBBS degree at the age of 22 years, can be understood because the age at which the person gets admitted to medical college is 17 years and it takes almost five years for one to obtain an MBBS degree (see Table 4.12).

Table 4.12

Doctors' Age-Group

Age (in Years)	*Government Hospital*	*Private Hospital*	*Total*
25–30	4 (18.18)	4 (18.18)	8 (36.36)
31–35	3 (13.63)	2 (9.09)	5 (22.73)
36–40	3 (13.63)	1 (4.55)	4 (18.18)
41–50	3 (13.63)	—	3 (13.63)
51 and above	—	2 (9.09)	2 (9.09)
Total	13 (59.09)	9 (40.91)	22 (100)

Figures in the bracket represent percentage.

Nativity of Doctors

The structural pattern of living either in rural or urban area gives us an understanding of the recruitment process of doctors in the medical profession. The rural-urban distinction is left to the judgement of the each respondent. Table 4.13 shows that 3 (13.63%) doctors are from rural area who are working in private hospital, whereas only one doctor is in government hospital who belongs to the rural area. Majority of, 12 (54.55%) doctors in government hospital belong to urban area. One may raise the point as to why there is a strong urban bias in the recruitment of the doctors when the proportion of urban in the total population of India is only 30 per cent. Venkatratnam (1979) argued that modern higher education attracts the urbanites first, as they are closer to the influence of institutions of higher learning.

Table 4.13

Nativity of Doctors

Nativity	*Government Hospital*	*Private Hospital*	*Total*
Rural	1 (4.55)	3 (13.63)	4 (18.18)
Urban	12 (54.55)	6 (27.28)	18 (81.82)
Total	13 (59.09)	9 (40.91)	22 (100)

Figures in the bracket represent percentage.

Type of Family of Doctors

Table 4.14 shows that 7 (31.82%) doctors who belong to joint family are all from rural origin, 15 (68.18%) who belonged to nuclear family, are of urban origin. Thus, it was clear that those are of urban origin belonged to nuclear family.

Table 4.14

Family Type of Doctors

Type of Family	*Government Hospital*	*Private Hospital*	*Total*
Joint	2 (9.09)	5 (22.73)	7 (31.82)
Nuclear	11 (50)	4 (18.18)	15 (68.18)
Total	13 (59.09)	9 (40.91)	22 (100)

Figures in the bracket represent percentage.

Marital Status of Doctors

Career decisions, particularly those involving movements from one place to another, may be heavily influenced by the obligations and restraints resulting from family responsibility at different stages of the family cycle. Out of the total sample, there are 19 (86.36%) married doctors and rest 3 (13.63%) are unmarried (see Table 4.15).

Table 4.15

Marital Status of Doctors

Marital Status	*Government Hospital*	*Private Hospital*	*Total*
Married	12 (54.54)	7 (31.82)	19 (86.36)
Unmarried	1 (4.54)	2 (9.09)	3 (13.63)
Total	13 (59.09)	9(40.91)	22 (100)

Figures in the bracket represent percentage.

Caste Background of Doctors

There have been several misgivings about the concepts of caste and class, and particularly with reference to their application to the understanding of Indian social reality. Here, we are not concerned with the concepts of caste and class but we are interested to understand a 'processual' system of social relations in the context of the recruitment of professionals in the field of medicine. This would provide an understanding of the dynamics of the caste system which also gives different class dimensions. We have adopted official classification for our analysis of caste background of doctors. We found that general castes account for 36.36 per cent of the total sample, other backward castes (OBC) for 54.55 per cent, and scheduled castes for 9.09 per cent. The largest representation is from other backward castes. There were only two scheduled caste doctors, both of whom are in government hospital. It is also found in Madan's study (1972: 84) that 15 per cent of doctors belong to clean upper castes, 82 per cent to clean middle castes, 3 per cent to clean lower castes and none to scheduled castes. Thus, we can view that people come in this profession from upper and middle castes which are economically better off and educationally and socially advanced as compared to lower and scheduled castes (see Table 4.16).

Table 4.16

Caste and Gender Category of Doctors

Caste/Category	*Government Hospital*		*Private Hospital*		*Total*
	Male	*Female*	*Male*	*Female*	
General*	—	3 (13.63)	2 (9.09)	3 (13.63)	8 (36.36)
OBC**	5 (22.73)	3 (13.63)	3 (13.63)	1 (4.55)	12 (54.55)
SC***	2 (9.09)	—	—	—	2 (9.09)
Total	7 (31.82)	6 (27.27)	5 (22.73)	4 (18.18)	22 (100)

Figures in the bracket represent percentage.

*General Category includes Brahmin, Bania, Khatri, Arora.
**Other Backward Caste includes Jat, Yadav, Khati, Kumhar, Panchal, Jat Sikh.
*** Scheduled Caste includes Chamar, Valmiki.

Educational Background of Doctors

Education brings changes in the society. It forms a social group on the basis of achievement which represents a social class. Therefore, educational background of doctors in terms of type of their degree and specialization helps to establish positions in the hierarchy of the social system and opens new avenues for mobility in the occupational structure of the society.

The data collected reveals that 8 (36.36%) respondents have higher specialization after MBBS, i.e. MD/MS and 31.82 per cent of doctors have MBBS as their basic degree for medical profession. There are five doctors who are serving in the private hospital and having their basic degree in Ayurveda which is called as BAMS (Bachelor of Ayurvedic Medicine and Surgery).

Table 4.17

Level of Education of Doctors

Level of Education	*Government Hospital*	*Private Hospital*	*Total*
BDS	2 (9.09)	—	2 (9.09)
BAMS	—	5 (22.73)	5 (22.73)
MBBS	7 (31.82)	—	7 (31.82)
MD/MS	4 (18.18)	4 (18.18)	8 (36.36)
Total	13 (59.09)	9 (40.91)	22 (100)

Figures in the bracket represent percentage.

Income of Doctors

Table 4.18 shows that majority, i.e. 31.82 per cent have their annual income between five to seven lakh rupees annually. Another 27.28 per cent of the doctors have their annual income more than nine lakh. There are only two doctors who have their annual income between three lakh to five lakh. There is a good possibility among doctors of not reporting their actual income.

Table 4.18

Income-Group of the Doctors

Annual Income-Group (in ₹)	*Government Hospital*	*Private Hospital*	*Total*
Less than three lakh	—	3 (13.63)	3 (13.63)
More than three lakh to five lakh	—	2 (9.09)	2 (9.09)
More than five to seven lakh	6 (27.28)	1 (4.55)	7 (31.82)
More than seven lakh to Nine lakh	2 (9.09)	2 (9.09)	4 (18.18)
Above Nine Lakh	5 (22.73)	1 (4.55)	6 (27.28)
Total	13 (59.09)	9 (40.91)	22 (100)

Figures in the bracket represent percentage.

The experience of doctors working in private and government hospitals is also seen in the context of their mobility from one health care facility to another. When there are fewer opportunities for the doctors in private sector, doctors prefer to serve in the same government hospital without shifting. However,

Table 4.19
Doctors' Experience in Hospital

Experience (in Years)	*Government Hospital*	*Private Hospital*	*Total*
Less than 5 years	7 (31.82)	4 (18.18)	11(50.0)
More than 5 year to 10 year	—	3 (13.63)	3 (13.63)
More than 10 year to 15 years	3 (13.63)	—	3 (13.63)
More than 15 year to 20 year	2 (9.09)	—	2 (9.09)
20 years and above	1 (4.55)	2 (9.09)	3 (13.63)
Total	13 (59.09)	9 (40.91)	22 (100)

Figures in the bracket represent percentage.

there are new corporate hospitals, clinics and other forms of health facilities coming up; therefore doctors have choice to move according to their convenience. Our study shows that maximum number of doctors, i.e. fifty per cent of doctors are having less than five years of their time period in the health facility where they are serving. Only 13.63 per cent of doctors are having more than 20 years of experience in the same hospital (see Table 4.19).

5

Health Rights of Patients and Ethics of Doctors

The idea of health and human rights as a subject of study is fairly new. Rights relating to autonomy, information, education, food and nutrition, association, equality and participation are integral and indivisible parts for the achievement of the highest attainable standard of health, just as the enjoyment of the 'right-to-health' is inseparable from all other rights.

Medical profession which is a noble profession has now become a business. Medical professionals often forget their responsibilities towards their patients and conduct their professional work without observing the code of ethics and thereby violate the rights of the patients. Growing incidences of malpractice and medical negligence of the patient results in the poor health or sometime in medical complications.

I

Health Rights of Patients

Before any treatment or investigation, patients have the right to a clear, concise explanation in lay terms of the proposed procedure and of any available alternative procedure. Where applicable the explanation shall incorporate information on risks, side-effects or after-effects, problems relating to recuperation, likelihood of success, risk of death, and whether the proposed procedure is to be administered by or in the presence of students. A patient may refuse any treatment or investigation.

If a patient is in hospital or any other health care facility, the patient shall, unless incapacitated, be consulted about any decision to discharge or transfer the patient to another facility. Where it is appropriate to a patient's condition or treatment, the patient shall be given advice about self-care, drug administration, special precautions which may be necessary or desirable, and the existence of special association, facilities, aids or appliances which may be of assistance. A patient's consent shall be required before any procedure is carried out. No patient shall be treated or examined without his or her consent. If a patient is incapacitated and delay would be dangerous, a doctor is entitled to carry out any necessary treatment or operation. A patient's written consent shall be required for the inclusion of a patient in any research. The patient shall be adequately informed of the aims, methods, anticipated benefits and potential hazards of the study and the discomfort it may entail. The patient shall be informed that he or she is free to withdraw his or her consent to participation at any time. To ensure that the informed consent is not obtained under duress or from a patient in a dependent relationship to the health professional, the informed consent shall be obtained by a health professional who is not engaged in the investigation and who is completely independent of the official relationship between the patient and the health professional.

Human life is precious and every person has a fundamental right to live with dignity. It is the duty of a welfare state to protect and develop the life of every citizen and to promote his rights to health and medical care. Right to medical care is important because it relates to the very existence of human life. Medical care is as essential as the other basic needs of a person like food, water, shelter and clothing. Every nation has evolved its own system of laws to ensure the health rights of its citizens. These laws aim to establish a humane system of health care based on the principles of equity, justice and efficiency. By emphasizing the rights of the citizens for proper health care the welfare government tries to enhance the welfare of its people so that they can live healthy and predictive lives.

Right to health and health care is also a fundamental right under Article 21 of the Constitution of India. This has also been emphasized by the Supreme Court of India in several obligations on the state to protect citizen's life from medical and other forms of negligence. Consumer Protection Act is applicable all over India but does not fall within the category of state-level health legislation.

Patients and their Diseases

At various times in the development of medicine, the causes of disease have been attributed to several phenomena. Even today, when some diseases are known to be caused by parasites, viruses and other bacteriological agents, the importance of environmental factors continue to get recognition. The genesis of the leading killers of diseases in India are because of inadequate supply of drinking water, low standards of environmental, sanitation and personal hygiene, road accidents, and mental tensions.

Table 5.1

Patients with their Type of Disease

Type of Disease	*Government Hospital*	*Private Hospital*	*Total*
Diseases related with medicine department like diabetes, blood pressure, acidity, pneumonia, malaria, dengue, asthma, chest/heart pain, diarrhea, etc.	19 (15.83)	43 (35.83)	62 (51.67)
Diseases related with surgery department like fractures in various body parts, surgery of uterus, hernia, stone removal in kidney, gallbladder, tumor, etc.	35 (29.17)	7 (5.83)	42 (35)
Tooth extraction, tooth setting, and other dental problems	2 (1.67)	—	2 (1.67)
Obstetrics and gynaecological disorders delivery of child, etc.	4 (3.33)	10 (8.33)	14 (11.67)
Total	60 (50)	60 (50)	120 (100)

Figures in the bracket represent percentage.

Table 5.1 shows that 43 (35.83%) patients who are suffering from diabetes, blood pressure, acidity, pneumonia, malaria, dengue, asthma, chest/heart pain, diarrhoea, etc. are seeking treatment in private hospital. There are 35 (29.17%) patients in government hospital suffering from fractures in various body parts, surgery of uterus, hernia, stone problem in kidney, gallbladder, tumour, etc. Patients do not want to go to private hospital for dental problem as it is a very costly affair and therefore in our study all patients are seeking their dental treatment from government hospital.

Concept of Health

Health development is the process of continuous progressive improvement of the health status of the population. Its product is rising level of human well-being not only by reduction in the burden of the disease but also by the attainment of positive, physical and mental health related to satisfactory economic functioning and social integration (Park and Park, 1990).

The concept of health cannot be seen in a narrow sense as a state of sheer absence of disease. It should be seen as a broad spectrum where health is viewed as integral well-being of the individuals (Mathur and Sharma, 1995). This holistic perception of health is well defined as 'health is state of complete physical, mental (or emotional) and social well being of a person and not mere absence of diseases' (WHO, 1988). The old ways of measuring the health status which included indices like mortality rates, particularly infant mortality rates and life expectancy seem to be reexamined today in the context of holistic perception of health. Presently health status indices include in addition to Infant Mortality Rate (IMR), variables such as drinking water, sanitation, morbidity, etc. (Cemper, 1984).

The operational definition of health says that it is 'a condition or quality of the human organism expressing the adequate functioning of the organism in given conditions, genetic or environmental. Maternal and child health refers to the promotive, preventive, curative and rehabilitative health care for mothers and children. It includes the sub-areas of maternal health, child health, family planning, school health, handicapped children in special, settings such as day care (Park and Park, 1990).

Poverty and ill health are interrelated. People become ill because they are poor; they also get poorer because they are ill. Inequality in the health statuses of people, particularly between developed and developing countries as well as within countries is politically, socially and economically unacceptable. Nearly 40 years after the Alma Ata declaration, health for all remains an elusive goal. Large disparities in health persist both within and between countries, health problems including parasitic and infectious diseases, nutritional deficiencies, birth complication, etc. are concentrated among the poor (WHO, 2001).

Table 5.2

Concept of Health as Viewed by the Patients

Concept of Health	*Government Hospital*	*Private Hospital*	*Total Response**
One who is energetic	35 (29.17)	40 (33.33)	75 (62.5)
Has good body build	33 (27.5)	34 (28.33)	67 (55.83)
Has all body organs functioning normally	46 (38.33)	52 (43.33)	98 (81.67)
Has a good appetite	44 (36.67)	49 (40.83)	93 (77.50)
Gets sound sleep	46 (38.33)	50 (41.67)	96 (80)
Able to work properly	36 (30)	38 (31.67)	74 (61.67)
Free from disease/illness	18 (15)	46 (38.33)	64 (53.33)

Figures in the bracket represent percentage.

*Multiple Responses.

Whenever we talk about health care, immediately it comes to our mind what is health and particularly how people view their health, what is the concept of health in their mind. The conception of the health will ultimately determine their way of thinking of remaining healthy as well as behaviour for seeking treatment. Although the response we get from the people can be subjective, but we have tried to ask them in such a manner which reflects the normative prescription of health in the society. To some respondents of our study, the term health does not connote anything obscure and elusive. The local equivalent for this is '*tandurasti*' which means right condition of the body. In the present study where we are trying to understand the health rights of the patients, it is utmost important to understand the conception of health in peoples' terminology. Table 5.2 shows their composite answers in certain categories. We recorded their answers in multiple response form as many respondents provided their concept of health in multidimensional form. Respondents are quite intelligent, as maximum number of answers, i.e. 98 (81.67%) responses are attributed to the normal functioning of the body which is also complementary to the scientific conception of health. Again 96 (80%) respondents attribute sound sleep as the necessary condition to be healthy. If one feels hungry and at the same time able to eat substantial amount of food is also regarded as healthy by 93 (77.50%) patients. Almost equal number of responses, i.e. sixty-two per cent viewed that good energy level as well as being able to work normally is also a sign of good health. However, 67 (55.83%) still feel that good body built is also reflection of the good health. Another 64 (53.33%) patients feel that a body free from any kind of disease and illness is a healthy body.

Table 5.3

Individual's Responsibility for His/Her Good Health as Viewed by the Patients

Individual's responsibility for his/her good health	*Nativity*		*Total Response**
	Rural	*Urban*	
Regular health check-up	26 (21.67)	16 (13.33)	42 (35)
Never ignore illness	32 (26.67)	34 (28.33)	66 (55)
Follow healthy lifestyles	53 (44.17)	28 (23.33)	81 (67.5)

Figures in the bracket represent percentage.

* Multiple Responses.

When we talk about their conception of good health, it is very important to understand their action pattern for remaining healthy. It also reflects their understanding of health issues while they seek treatment and also in terms of their health rights. Table 5.3 shows that majority of respondent's, i.e. 81 (67.5%) view that it is important to follow healthy lifestyles and only 42 (35%) patients feel that each individual should go for regular health check-up for his/her good health. Majority of the, 81 (67.5%), patients believe in following healthy lifestyle for good health and they reported that it is the individual's responsibility to remain healthy. Here it is very interesting to note that more than eighty per cent feel that in absence of healthy lifestyle, diseases emerge and therefore, taking it as a individual's responsibility, lifestyle can be improved upon.

Admission into Hospital

Table 5.4 shows that maximum number of patients, i.e. 54 (45%) who are seeking treatment in government or private hospital have previously tried ayurvedic treatment. Nearly forty-four per cent patients have just ignored their illness and therefore, they did not take any treatment before coming here. Around 40 per cent of the patients visited *Jhola chap* doctors who do not have any proper degree in the medical science. And 12 (10%) patients who are seeking treatment in government hospital had previously visited the subcentre, primary health centre, community health centre, and other government general hospital. There are only 21 (17.5%) patients who did not go anywhere and directly came here for the treatment.

Table 5.4

Visit of Patients before taking Treatment in Government/Private Hospital

Visit of patient before hospitalization	*Government Hospital*	*Private Hospital*	*Total Response**
Government Subcentre, PHC, CHC, General Hospital, etc.	12 (10)	19 (15.83)	31 (25.83)
Private Hospital/Clinics	3 (2.5)	17 (14.17)	20 (16.67)
Ayurvedic Treatment	22 (18.33)	32 (26.67)	54 (45)
Ignore illness	25 (20.83)	27 (22.5)	52 (43.33)
Jhola chap Doctor	23 (19.17)	25 (20.83)	48 (40)
Did not go anywhere	7 (5.83)	14 (11.67)	21 (17.5)

Figures in the bracket represent percentage.

* Multiple Responses.

As soon as one's body gives signals of improper functioning, one feels that something is wrong and which is beyond his/her capacity to manage at home. In majority of the cases people do their own remedies to get well, if it is in their purview, otherwise they go to the health care facility. What are the symptoms or how they realized that they are suffering from some illness? These responses are which we collected during our fieldwork and categorized them into certain meaningful categories.

Problems in Admission in Hospital

Table 5.5 shows that 19 (15.83%) patients in government hospital faced problem in admission process, whereas only 1.67 patients faced problem in admission in private hospital. It means seeking treatment in government hospital is a cumbersome process.

Table 5.5

Patient's Admission Process in Hospital

Problem Faced by Patients in Admission Process	*Government Hospital*	*Private Hospital*	*Total*
Yes	19 (15.83)	2 (1.67)	21 (17.5)
No	41 (34.17)	58 (48.33)	99 (82.5)
Total	60 (50)	60 (50)	120 (100)

Figures in the bracket represent percentage.

Around 21 (17.5%) patients who faced problem while getting admission into hospital reported that doctors just ignore their seriousness of illness. Furthermore, 10 (47.62%) experienced that doctors are more interested in referring them to some other health care facility. Nearly ten per cent patients reported that their illnesses are not serious in nature therefore, doctors also did not take interest in admitting them (see Table 5.6).

Table 5.6

Nature of Problems Faced by Patient in Admission Process

Nature of Problems in Admission Process	*Government Hospital*	*Private Hospital*	*Total Response**
Ignored by Doctors	18 (85.71)	—	18 (85.71)
Not so serious illness, therefore doctor ignored	1 (4.76)	1 (4.76)	2 (9.52)
Doctors are interested in referring to the other facility	9 (42.86)	1 (4.76)	10 (47.62)

Figures in the bracket represent percentage.

* Multiple Responses.

Realization of Illness by Patients

A symptom is any subjective evidence of disease, while a sign is any objective evidence of disease. Therefore, a symptom is a phenomenon that is experienced by the individual affected by the disease, while a sign is a phenomenon that can be detected by someone other than the individual affected by the disease. For example, anxiety, pain, and fatigue are all symptoms. In contrast, a bloody nose is a sign of injured blood vessels in the nose that can be detected by a doctor, a nurse, or another observer. Health care professionals use symptoms and signs as clues that can help to determine the most likely diagnosis when illness occurs. Symptoms and signs are also used to compose a list of the possible diagnoses. This listing is referred to as the differential diagnosis. The differential diagnosis is the basis from which initial tests are ordered to narrow down the possible diagnostic options and choose initial treatments. Table 5.7 shows that majority, 110 (91.66%), of patients replied that they felt pain in different parts of body. Another 67 (55.83%) felt sleeping disorder, whereas 50 (41.67%) reported that they did not feel like having food or were in a state of loss of appetite. A significant number of respondents, i.e. 44 (36.67%) felt disorder in their urine system in terms of increased frequency of urine discharge, swollen bladder and pain while urinating, etc. Nearly fifty-five per cent felt weakness in their body and 28.33 per cent reported problem of bleeding (it was applicable mostly in case of female patients). There were 21 (17.5%) patients who reported of frequent vomiting.

Table 5.7

Realization of Illness felt by the Patients

Illness realization	*Government Hospital*	*Private Hospital*	*Total Response**
Sleep Disorder	19 (15.83)	48 (40)	67 (55.83)
Loss of Appetite	16 (13.33)	34 (28.33)	50 (41.67)
Pain in body	52 (43.33)	58 (48.33)	110 (91.66)
Weakness in body	16 (13.33)	40 (33.33)	56 (46.67)
Frequent Vomiting	10 (8.33)	11 (9.17)	21 (17.5)
Swollen Urine bladder/ frequent urine problem	14 (11.67)	30 (25)	44 (36.67)
Bleeding problem	32 (26.67)	2 (1.67)	34 (28.33)

Figures in the bracket represent percentage.

* Multiple Responses.

Prescription of Doctors

When one enters into the hospital or in any other health care facility, one is supposed to follow the prescription of doctors to get well soon. This is also explained by Parsons (1951) in terms of sick role. Doctor is a specialized professional and at the same time he is competent to prescribe treatment on the basis of his specialized knowledge and skill. Doctor is a provider of health care and patient is in the role of receiving of health care from the doctor. It may be in the form of fee directly paid by the patients in the private hospital or indirectly wherein government is paying for its citizens to the doctors in government hospitals. Just to see how people follow the prescription of doctors in their process of treatment, we asked our respondents to give their answers about how they follow the exact prescription of doctors during the process of treatment or do they simply ignore it.

Table 5.8

Patients Following Treatment Prescribed by Doctors

Following Prescription of Doctors	*Government Hospital*	*Private Hospital*	*Total*
Yes	14 (11.67)	30 (25)	44 (36.67)
No	46 (38.33)	30 (25)	76 (63.33)
Total	60 (50)	60 (50)	120 (100)

Figures in the bracket represent percentage.

Table 5.8 shows that 76 (63.33%) patients do not follow the treatment prescribed by the doctors. There are only 44 (36.67%) patients who follow the treatment prescribed by the doctors. Further, we asked our respondents as to reply why they did not follow doctors' prescription. The answers are recorded in multiple forms.

Table 5.9

Causes for not Following the Prescription of Doctors by the Patients

Causes for not Following the Prescription	*Government Hospital*	*Private Hospital*	*Total Response**
Due to poor economic condition	29 (38.16)	11 (14.47)	40 (52.63)
Now cured	32 (42.1)	29 (38.16)	61 (80.26)
Due to busy lifestyle	36 (47.37)	23 (30.26)	59 (77.63)
Forget to take medicine in time	34 (44.74)	21(27.63)	55 (72.37)
When visit to doctors and do not find we just leave the prescription	17 (22.37)	5 (6.58)	22 (28.95)

Figures in the bracket represent percentage.

* Multiple Responses.

Table 5.9 shows that majority of patients 59 (77.63%) accept that they do not follow the prescription of doctors due to busy lifestyle. Around 34 (44.74%) patients accept that they skip the prescription of doctors as they forget to take medicine or other advice on time. Another 52.63 per cent replied that because of their poor economic condition they are unable to continue with the treatment. Maximum number of patients, i.e. 61 (80.26%) replied that when they feel that they are cured they immediately stop the treatment ignoring the prescription of treatment for further wellness. Little less than thirty per cent feel that as and when they go to the doctor to consult and if they do not find that doctor who had earlier prescribed the treatment, they leave the treatment midway.

Table 5.10

Reading of Doctor's Prescription by Patients

Reading of Doctor's Prescription	*Government Hospital*	*Private Hospital*	*Total*
Yes	3 (2.5)	10 (8.33)	13 (10.83)
No	57 (47.5)	50 (41.67)	107 (89.17)
Total	60 (50)	60 (50)	120 (100)

Figures in the bracket represent percentage.

Table 5.10 shows that only 13 (10.83%) patients read the prescription given by doctors. Majority of patients, 107 (89.17%) in government and private hospitals do not read the prescription of doctors.

Table 5.11

Pressure of Patients on Doctors for Immediate Relief

Pressure of Patients for Immediate Relief	*Government Hospital*	*Private Hospital*	*Total*
Yes	7 (5.83)	10 (8.33)	17 (14.17)
No	53 (44.17)	50 (41.67)	103 (85.83)
Total	60 (50)	60 (50)	120 (100)

Figures in the bracket represent percentage.

Table 5.11 shows that 10 (8.33%) patients in private hospital pressurized the doctor for immediate relief. There are 53

(44.17%) patients in government hospital who do not say anything regarding the treatment process.

Table 5.12

Causes for not Pressurizing Doctors for Fast Relief

Causes for not Pressurize	*Government Hospital*	*Private Hospital*	*Total Response**
Doctor is more expert in his profession	36 (34.95)	47 (45.63)	83 (80.58)
We should not interfere with treatment process	13 (12.62)	26 (25.24)	39 (37.86)
Some diseases take time to get cured	11 (10.68)	13 (12.62)	24 (23.30)

Figures in the bracket represent percentage.

* Multiple Responses.

Furthermore, we asked our respondents to give the reasons, as to why they do not want to pressurize doctors for immediate relief. They very wisely replied in multiple forms. As many as 83 (80.58%) feel that they are not competent and doctor is specialized in his profession and another 39 (37.86%) replied that they do not want to interfere in the process of treatment prescribed by the doctor. More than one-fifth of the respondents feel that the treatment process of some diseases is long, therefore, it take its own time (see Table 5.12).

Cost of Treatment

Health care treatment is not only concerned with physical pain, social stigma, exemption from social roles but it also has economic aspects. Giving priority to money reflects the attitude of people in the capitalistic society. It has been argued in many empirical studies that people spend lot of money for the treatment for their family members which sometimes results into indebtedness. Loan for illness is an important cause of indebtedness in Indian society. People still care for their loved ones. We recorded peoples' attitude for spending money for the treatment of their family members.

In a bid to maximize profits, there is a tendency to overtreat the patient. This is possible under two circumstances: first, the patient's level of ignorance about his disease is absolutely very high and second the patient is completely dependent on the doctor. In many countries, iatrogenic illness arising out of the medical care process itself is a major problem and there is a widespread perception that many of the operations should not have been performed. Too much dependency on the part of the patient is indeed a necessary evil. The patient has no right to know about the medicine used, its quality and also the quality of the care being taken by the doctor. The cost and quality of care vary from doctor to doctor and also from hospital to hospital. But the poor patient has no way to determine all these crucial issues in detail before beginning the treatment protocol. It is also difficult within the system of bounded rationality for the patients to make proper choices before or during the period of treatment and more often than not, things are forced on to patients. The doctor can compel the patient to buy more medicine than what is necessary and advise him to come more frequently for a check-up. All this creates a supply-induced demand. In order to recover the heavy overhead costs of private hospitals, the innocent patients are often asked to undergo tests which are not really warranted and whose cost for the patients is extremely high (Fuchs, 1981).

Table 5.13

Patients and their Worries about Medical Care Cost

Cause of no worry about Medical Care Cost	*Government Hospital*	*Private Hospital*	*Total Response**
Life is more important than money	22 (18.33)	31 (25.83)	53 (44.17)
Good economic condition	11 (9.17)	20 (16.67)	31 (25.83)
Getting Free treatment because they are from Below Poverty Line	14 (11.67)	—	14 (11.67)
Ex-Servicemen (Reimbursement)	1 (.83)	6 (5)	7 (5.83)
Disease also part of life	14 (11.67)	27 (22.5)	41 (34.17)

Figures in the bracket represent percentage.

* Multiple Responses.

Table 5.13 shows that majority of patients, 53 (44.17%) are more worried about the life of their loved ones than the money, and 31 (25.83%) respondents replied that they do not have any economic problem, therefore they are not worried about the cost of treatment. There is no patient in private hospital who is worried about their economic problem. Around 14 (11.67%) reported that they are not worried about the cost of treatment as they are getting free treatment because they are from below poverty line, whereas 7 (5.83%) reported that they are covered under the reimbursement scheme, therefore they are not worried about the cost of treatment. Surprisingly, 41 (34.17%) take it otherwise that disease and illness are also part of life, therefore during the course of life one has to spend for the treatment also.

Patients' Awareness of Treatment

Generally, a patient is aware about his illness, pain or discomfort which he/she experiences during his illness. However, many of the patients are not at all aware of their course of treatment, medicines and their diagnosis. To know people's awareness about the patients' level of awareness, we have tried to ask them about the awareness of expiry date of medicines.

Table 5.14

Patients' Awareness of Expiry Date of Medicines

Level of Education	*Government Hospital*		*Private Hospital*		*Total*
	Yes	*No*	*Yes*	*No*	
Illiterate	—	20 (16.67)	—	18 (15)	38 (31.67)
Primary	—	9 (7.5)	1 (.83)	5 (4.17)	15 (12.5)
Middle	1 (.83)	13 (10.83)	1 (.83)	4 (3.33)	19 (15.83)
Matriculation	—	6 (5)	2 (1.67)	2 (1.67)	10 (8.33)
10+2	3 (2.5)	5 (4.17)	5 (4.17)	2 (1.67)	15 (12.5)
BA/BEd	2 (1.67)	1 (.83)	11 (9.17)	5 (4.17)	19 (15.83)
MA/MSc	—	—	3 (2.5)	1 (.83)	4 (3.33)
Total	6 (5)	54 (45)	23 (19.17)	37 (30.83)	120 (100)

Figures in the bracket represent percentage.

Table 5.14 shows that 31.67 per cent patients cannot read and write; therefore, obviously they do not read the expiry date of medicines. Further, they do not ask any other person who is literate to take note of the expiry date of medicines. There are 13 (10.83%) patients in government hospital and 4 (3.33%) patients in private hospital who are middle standard educated but do not take the note of expiry date of medicines. There are 13 (10.83%) graduate patients who note the expiry date of medicines. It is shocking to note that even postgraduate patients in private hospital ignore expiry date of medicines. There are only one quarter of respondents, who note the date of expiry of medicines before taking it. It shows that the awareness about reading of expiry date increases with the level of education.

Table 5.15

Reasons for not Reading the Expiry Date of Medicines

Reasons for not Reading the Expiry Date	*Government Hospital*	*Private Hospital*	*Total Responses**
Due to unawareness	38 (41.76)	22 (24.17)	60 (65.93)
Confidence on chemist	27 (29.67)	24 (26.37)	51 (56.04)
Regular supply and demand of medicine	28 (30.77)	21 (23.07)	49 (53.85)
No time to check	6 (6.59)	5 (5.49)	11 (12.08)
Medicine in broken packet	27 (29.67)	21 (23.07)	48 (52.75)

Figures in the bracket represent percentage.

*Multiple responses

All the 91 (75.83%) respondents who replied that they do not bother to read the expiry date of medicines mentioned certain reasons for not taking care of expiry of medicines. However, out of 91, 38 (31.67%) are illiterate; therefore they did not give reason. 60 (65.93%) respondents mentioned that they are not aware of expiry of medicines. Another 51 (56.04%) replied that they have full confidence in chemist and he himself will not give any expired medicine. Around 49 (53.85%) replied that the shop from which they buy medicine is a very popular shop; therefore it has a regular demand and supply of medicines. Thus, there is no question of expiry date. Only 11 (12.08%) replied that they do not have time to check the expiry date, and 48 (52.75%) replied that they get medicine in broken packets, therefore, unable to read it. Table 5.15 shows that 66 per cent patients in government hospital and private hospital are unable to read the expiry date of medicines because they are not aware. Around 27 (29.67%) patients in government hospital have confidence in chemist, so they do not read the expiry date of medicines. Only 5 (5.49%) patients in private hospital do not have time to check the expiry date of medicines.

Health Rights of Patients

The present chapter focuses on the understanding of health right issues in context of knowledge of health rights, manifestation of patient's rights, publicity of health rights, patients' responsibility towards health rights, informed consent, satisfaction from treatment, responses for equal health rights, medical negligence, sharing of information about treatment, forms of malpractice and suggestions for improvement of health right information. We will discuss below the above mentioned issues.

Table 5.16

Knowledge of Health Rights Among Patients and Literacy Level

Level of Education	*Yes*	*No*	*Total*
Illiterate	1 (.83)	37 (30.83)	38 (31.67)
Primary	2 (1.67)	13 (10.83)	15 (12.5)
Middle	3 (2.5)	16 (13.33)	19 (15.83)
Matriculation	3 (2.5)	7 (5.83)	10 (8.33)
10+2	7 (5.83)	8 (6.67)	15 (12.5)
BA/B.Ed	16 (13.33)	3 (2.5)	19 (15.83)
MA/MSc	4 (3.33)	—	4 (3.33)
Total	36 (30)	84 (70)	120 (120)

Figures in the bracket represent percentage.

Table 5.16 shows that 37 (30.83%) illiterate patients are not at all aware of their health rights. Only 3 (2.5%) patients who are middle pass have the knowledge of health rights. Whereas, 16 (13.33%) graduate patients have the knowledge of health rights. All the four patients who are postgraduates mentioned that they have knowledge of health rights. On further probing about the knowledge of health rights, we received multiple responses.

Every hospital, big or small requires setting up of a well organized emergency unit, because the image of hospital mainly depends upon the quality and type of treatment a hospital can provide to a patient suffering from any medical or surgical complications, requiring immediate care. Emergency Department of a hospital is a part of hospital to which persons injured in road accidents or those suffering from serious complications are taken for urgent treatment. It is in this context that the Emergency Department of the hospital is often the point of major public impact, even more than the out-patient department, providing every important service and at the same time being the most vulnerable to criticism and censure. The department is meant to provide round the clock, immediate diagnosis and best possible treatment for illness of emergency nature and injuries from accidents (Balaraman, 1990).

Table 5.17

Patients' Understanding of Health Rights

Meaning of Health Rights	*Government Hospital*	*Private Hospital*	*Total Response**
Right to live with dignity	8 (6.67)	17 (14.17)	25 (20.83)
Government's responsibility to provide health services	9 (7.5)	23 (19.17)	32 (26.67)
Free health services	8 (6.67)	9 (7.5)	17 (14.17)
Well diagnosed treatment	5 (4.17)	21 (17.5)	26 (21.67)
Emergent treatment of health problem	7 (5.83)	20 (16.67)	27 (22.5)

Figures in the bracket represent percentage.

* Multiple Responses.

Table 5.17 shows that 17 (14.17%) patients in private hospital understand the meaning of health right as the right to live with dignity. Around 32 (26.67%) patients understand health right as government's responsibility to provide health service. Whereas, 17 (14.17%) patients replied that health rights means to get free health services. Another 26 (21.67%) reported that health right means very well diagnosed form of treatment. Similarly, 27 (22.5%) replied that getting treatment in the emergency/casualty in government hospital is health right.

Table 5.18

Manifestation of Patient's Health Right viewed by Patients

Manifestation of Patient's Right	*Government Hospital*	*Private Hospital*	*Total Response**
To receive treatment	55 (45.83)	57 (47.5)	112 (93.33)
Emergency Medical Care irrespective of anything	31 (25.83)	34 (28.33)	65 (54.17)
Treatment without any discrimination	25 (20.83)	44 (36.67)	69 (57.5)
To get the benefit of health facilities	26 (21.67)	25 (20.83)	51 (42.5)
Right to information	9 (7.5)	14 (11.67)	23 (19.17)
Right to informed consent	5 (4.17)	16 (13.33)	21 (17.5)
Confidentiality	5 (4.17)	14 (11.67)	19 (15.83)

Figures in the bracket represent percentage.

* Multiple Responses.

Table 5.18 shows that majority of patients, 112 (93.33%) in government and private hospitals think that patients' right is to receive treatment. Only 14 (15.83%) patients replied that every patient has a right of confidentiality of his/her treatment, which means that doctor is not supposed to disclose his/her disease to others. A good number of patients, i.e. 66 (55%) replied that as and when there is an emergency of treatment, it should be given immediately without asking for any fee or question, whether in government or private health facility. Another significant number of patients view health right in terms of adequate health care. However, crucial elements of right to health care are not given much importance by patients as only nearly 20 per cent replied that they have a right to ask about the process of treatment, and another 21 patients reported that they have right to informed consent. Informed consent means without their knowledge doctor cannot do any surgery on their body. Almost seventy patients feel that there should be no discrimination in treatment.

Views on Publicity of Health Rights

Table 5.19 shows that majority of patients, i.e. 117 (97%) have gathered information of health rights from news papers and television. Another 77 (64.17%) patients in government and private hospitals had collected information about health right from hospitals only where they were admitted. About 36 (30%) patients in government hospitals have taken the help of neighbours for health right information. Around 19 (15.83%) patients of private hospital gathered information from the posters displayed at various public places. Whereas, 67 (55.83%) patients have knowledge about health right information which they received from their family members.

Any society comes to know about the information from the society itself, although there are different modes through which they can accumulate the information. We asked our informants as to what they think is best for the dissemination of information of health rights in the society.

Table 5.19

Source of Health Right Information

Source of Information	*Government Hospital*	*Private Hospital*	*Total Response**
After getting admitted in the hospital	48 (40)	29 (24.17)	77 (64.17)
Family	44 (36.67)	23 (19.17)	67 (55.83)
Friends	33 (27.7)	16 (13.33)	49 (40.83)
Neighbours	36 (30)	14 (11.67)	50 (41.67)
Relatives	16 (13.33)	13 (10.83)	29 (24.17)
Books	2 (1.67)	3 (2.5)	5 (4.17)
Posters in hospitals	17 (14.17)	19 (15.83)	36 (30)
Newspapers	31 (25.83)	23 (19.17)	54 (45)
TV	38 (31.67)	25 (20.83)	63 (52.5)

Figures in the bracket represent percentage.

* Multiple Responses.

Majority of patients, i.e. 55 per cent believed that it is necessary to disseminate information about health rights in the society particularly through text books in school and colleges. Only four patients replied that there is no need of dissemination of information of health rights. However, fifty patients replied that they do not know how to disseminate information of health rights (see Table 5.20).

Table 5.20

Dissemination of Information of Health Right

Response	*Government Hospital*	*Private Hospital*	*Total*
Yes	27 (22.5)	39 (32.5)	66 (55)
No	4 (3.33)	—	4 (3.33)
Don't Know	29 (24.17)	21 (17.5)	50 (41.67)
Total	60 (50)	60 (50)	120 (100)

Figures in the bracket represent percentage.

Patient's Responsibility towards Rights

Generally people talk about health rights and they tend to forget their duties/responsibilities. Rights and duties go together. If you ask for rights, duties come attached with them. Therefore, it is pertinent to ask about the responsibilities of patients when they seek treatment from the doctors.

When we asked about the patients' responsibility during the process of treatment, all patients replied some or other form of responsibilities in the form of multiple answers. Majority of the patients, i.e. 110 (91.66%) replied that it is the duty of the patient to give the fee to the doctor which is agreed upon or which is written on the board. Another 78 (65%) patients feel that their responsibility lies in giving respect to the doctors. Many empirical studies have confirmed that people still equate doctor with god; therefore, in our study also people feel that responsibility of patients is to give respect to doctors. Nearly fifty per cent patients feel that their responsibility lies in cooperation with the doctors in the treatment process, which has also been explained by Parsons in his conception of sick role. Increasing number of episodes of violence cases reported in the hospitals by patients are opposed by 31 (25.83%) patients (see Table 5.21).

Table 5.21

Patient's Responsibilities towards Doctor

Patient's Responsibilities	*Government Hospital*	*Private Hospital*	*Total Response**
Provide his/her health related information	25 (20.83)	36 (30)	61 (50.83)
Cooperate with doctor's examination process	26 (21.67)	32 (26.67)	58 (48.33)
Maintaining hygiene in the hospital	17 (14.17)	25 (20.83)	42 (35)
Pay agreed fees	52 (43.33)	58 (48.33)	110 (91.66)
Respect the dignity of doctor	36 (30)	42 (35)	78 (65)
Never resort to violence	13 (10.83)	18 (15)	31 (25.83)

Figures in the bracket represent percentage.

* Multiple Responses.

Informed Consent and Health Rights

Informed consent is one of the central concepts of present-day medical ethics. The right of the patient to make decision about their health has been enshrined in legal and ethical statements in our code of ethics. It states that:

> The patient has the right to self-determination, to make free decisions himself/herself. The physician will inform the patient

of the consequences of his/her decisions. A mentally competent adult patient has the right to give or withhold consent to any diagnostic procedure or therapy. The patient has the right to the information necessary to make his/her decisions. The patient should understand clearly, what the purpose of any test or treatment is, what the result would imply, and what would be the implications of withholding consent.

With the increasing level of knowledge among people in the society, it becomes necessary that people should have the knowledge of their treatment. When people have knowledge of their treatment, automatically they can also question the line of treatment and it becomes easier for them to give consent for the treatment.

Table 5.22

Patient's Knowledge about the Consent of Treatment

Knowledge of Consent	*Government Hospital*	*Private Hospital*	*Total*
Yes	11 (9.17)	28 (23.33)	39 (32.5)
No	49 (40.83)	32 (26.67)	81 (67.5)
Total	60 (50)	60 (50)	120 (100)

Figures in the bracket represent percentage.

In our study 81 (67.5%) patients have no knowledge about consent of treatment. These patients replied that they do not understand the complexity of treatment and only doctor is competent enough to take decision for their treatment. However, 39 (32.5%) patients reported that they are competent enough to give their consent for the treatment (see Table 5.22).

Satisfaction/Dissatisfaction of Patients from Treatment

How, then, do we know whether people are satisfied or dissatisfied with the consultation, with the treatment and with their doctor in general. Satisfaction and dissatisfaction are concepts which, like expectations, are difficult to operationalize in research. Abrams (1968) has argued that this is a matter of the refinement of questioning techniques. We would suggest that it is because of the fluctuating nature of people's feelings about their encounters with doctors. What may be seen as satisfactory in one context may be seen as unsatisfactory in another. For example, one person describes her doctor as being good with children and explained that she was always happy with his treatment of her son, only to criticize that same concern over her child's health when the doctor made an unrequested home visit which she considered to be unnecessary.

Table 5.23

Patient's Response about Satisfaction from Treatment

Satisfaction from Treatment	*Government Hospital*	*Private Hospital*	*Total*
Yes	38 (31.67)	43 (35.83)	81 (67.5)
No	22 (18.33)	17 (14.17)	39 (32.5)
Total	60 (50)	60 (50)	120 (100)

Figures in the bracket represent percentage.

Satisfaction from the treatment not only helps in the healing process but also provide good interaction and relationship between doctors and patients. To know the satisfaction from the treatment, we asked our respondents if they were satisfied with the treatment they were receiving from the hospital. Majority of them, i.e. 81 (67.5%) reported that they are satisfied with the treatment they were receiving from the hospital. There is variation in terms of satisfaction in government and private hospital. More number of patients in private hospital are satisfied with the treatment as compared to government hospital. Only 39 (32.5%) patients are not satisfied with the treatment (see Table 5.23).

Table 5.24

Patients' Satisfaction with Doctor's Behaviour

Satisfaction with behaviour of doctors	*Government Hospital*	*Private Hospital*	*Total*
Yes	39 (32.5)	49 (40.83)	88 (73.33)
No	21 (17.5)	11 (9.17)	32 (26.67)
Total	60 (50)	60 (50)	120 (100)

Figures in the bracket represent percentage.

Nearly seventy per cent of patients are satisfied with doctor's behaviour. However, 32 (26.67%) are not satisfied with doctor's behaviour. The patients who are not satisfied with doctor's behaviour are more from government hospital (see Table 5.24).

Table 5.25

Patients' Dissatisfaction with the Behaviour of Doctors

Causes of Dissatisfaction	*Government Hospital*	*Private Hospital*	*Total Responses**
Not paying equal attention to all	16 (50)	3 (9.37)	19 (59.37)
Rude behaviour	11 (34.37)	10 (31.25)	21 (65.62)
Do not share line of treatment	9 (28.12)	1 (3.12)	10 (31.25)

Figures in the bracket represent percentage.

* Multiple Responses.

Further, the dissatisfaction from the behaviour of doctors is reported in terms of their rude behaviour, discrimination in treatment and doctors not sharing the line of treatment. Majority of patients, i.e. 19 (59.37) feel that doctors do not pay equal attention to all. They are biased towards their own kin, caste, relatives, etc. (see Table 5.25).

Similarly, we also asked about their satisfaction from the treatment process.

Table 5.26

Patients' Satisfaction from Treatment

Causes of Satisfaction	*Government Hospital*	*Private Hospital*	*Total Responses**
Proper care	11 (13.58)	30 (37.03)	41 (50.62)
All tests available	7 (8.64)	27 (33.33)	34 (41.97)
Test report on time	4 (4.93)	21 (25.93)	25 (30.86)
Nominal charges	18 (22.22)	16 (19.75)	34 (41.97)

Figures in the bracket represent percentage.

* Multiple Responses.

Equal number of patients, i.e. 34 (41.97%) reported that they are getting proper care in the hospital at nominal charges. However, the level of satisfaction in terms of proper care is high in private hospital as compared to government hospital. Satisfaction in terms of diagnostic tests and timely reports of tests is more in case of private hospitals as compared to government hospitals (see Table 5.26).

Overall dissatisfaction with the facility of health care in government and private hospital is reported by the patients for multiple reasons. These vary from shortage of doctors, beds, nurses and paramedical staff. Another important cause of dissatisfaction comes from the poor hygiene in hospital and dirty bedsheets. Most of the diagnostic tests are delayed as machines are not found in order and sometimes they are faulty also. That is why patients have doubt on the diagnostic tests done by the hospital staff. Some of them also reported doctor's biasness in treatment. The patients are not treated with dignity and respect.

Table 5.27

Patients' Dissatisfaction from Hospital Services

Causes of Dissatisfaction	*Government Hospital*	*Private Hospital*	*Total Responses**
Due to shortage of doctors	22 (56.41)	—	22 (56.41)
No proper care by doctors	19 (48.72)	7 (17.95)	26 (66.67)
Due to shortage of ward staff	18 (46.15)	10 (25.64)	28 (71.79)
Due to shortage of beds for the patients	16 (41.02)	—	16 (41.02)
Not having proper medical knowledge	13 (33.33)	7 (17.95)	20 (51.28)
Insufficient paramedical staff	20 (51.28)	16 (41.02)	36 (92.31)
High cost of treatment	—	17 (43.59)	17 (43.59)
Delay in diagnostic tests	21 (53.85)	3 (7.69)	24 (61.54)
Doubt on diagnostic tests done by hospital	11 (28.20)	7 (17.95)	18 (46.15)
Due to shortage of diagnostic tools	5 (12.82)	3 (7.69)	8 (20.51)
Discrimination in care	22 (56.41)	8 (20.51)	30 (76.92)
Failing to treat the patient with dignity or respect	22 (56.41)	5 (12.82)	27 (69.23)
Dirty bedsheets	21 (53.85)	9 (23.08)	30 (76.92)
Poor sanitation and hygiene	19 (48.72)	12 (30.77)	31 (79.49)

Figures in the bracket represent percentage.

* Multiple Responses.

Table 5.28

Patient's Response for Equal Rights for Health Care

Response for Equal Rights for health care	*Government Hospital*	*Private Hospital*	*Total*
Yes	17 (14.17)	15 (12.5)	32 (26.67)
No	43 (35.83)	45 (37.5)	88 (73.33)
Total	60 (50)	60 (50)	120 (100)

Figures in the bracket represent percentage.

We asked our respondents to give their views about the equality of health rights. Majority of the patients, i.e. 88 (73.33%) replied that there is a discrepancy in realization of health rights. However, 32 (26.67%) opined that there are equal health rights for all irrespective of their caste, class, age, gender, education level (see Table 5.28). Further, we asked as to why there are no equal health rights for all. They replied in multiple response form.

Table 5.29

Causes of Unequal Health Rights

Causes of Unequal Health Rights	*Government Hospital*	*Private Hospital*	*Total Responses**
Health right only for rich people	38 (43.18)	43 (48.86)	81 (92.04)
Health right only for people with higher reach	36 (40.91)	23 (26.14)	59 (67.04)

Figures in the bracket represent percentage.

* Multiple Responses.

81 (92.04%) patients feel that health rights are only meant for rich people and another 59 (67.04%) opined that health rights are exercised by people with good connections (see Table 5.29).

Medical Negligence and Health Right

It is very difficult to understand the concept of medical negligence particularly by the layman who is not aware of the complexity of medical treatment. It is a highly technical and scientific area of investigation. However, we asked our patients to give their views about medical negligence in simple terms.

Table 5.30

Patient's Understanding of Medical Negligence

Understanding of Medical Negligence	Government Hospital		Private Hospital		Total
	Rural	Urban	Rural	Urban	
Yes	6 (5)	11 (9.17)	10 (8.33)	11 (9.17)	38 (31.67)
No	33 (27.5)	10 (8.33)	30 (25)	9 (7.5)	82 (68.33)
Total	39 (32.5)	21 (17.5)	40 (33.33)	20 (16.67)	120 (100)

Figures in the bracket represent percentage.

Our study also confirms that because of the complexity in understanding of medical negligence, majority of the respondents, i.e. 82 (68.33%) reported that they do not understand the medical negligence committed by doctors. However, 38 (31.67%) stated that they do understand the medical negligence. Urban patients are more aware of medical negligence as compared to patients who come from rural area.

Sharing of Information about Treatment

It is necessary to share the information regarding the cost of treatment, benefits of treatment, and risk in particular treatment process from health right perspective. In the normal circumstances, it is expected that doctor should share the information regarding the cost of treatment, risk involved in the particular treatment and consequences of the treatment. However, in our study 65 (54.17%) patients are not ready to accept that they should have information regarding the treatment process and risk involved. Little more than forty-five per cent do feel that they should have complete information regarding the cost of treatment, consequences of treatment and risk involved in particular treatment (see Table 5.31).

Table 5.31

Patients' Opinion about Sharing of Information about Treatment

Patients' Opinion about Sharing of Information about Treatment	Government Hospital	Private Hospital	Total
Yes	26 (21.67)	29 (24.17)	55 (45.83)
No	34 (28.33)	31 (25.83)	65 (54.17)
Total	60 (50)	60 (50)	120 (100)

Figures in the bracket represent percentage.

Suggestions for Improvement of Health Rights Information

Patients' cognition and understanding of health is also reflected in their suggestions which they gave for improving the health rights understanding and their implementation. Maximum number of patients, i.e. 95 (79.17%) replied that there should be display of patients' right at every gate of the hospital so that people can easily read them. Another 82 (68.33%) opined that every section, whether OPD or Indoor Care should have information about health rights. Nearly fifty per cent of the patients feel that media can play a significant role in disseminating information about health rights. Nearly 40 per cent of the patients reported that there should be inclusion of chapter on health rights in the text books at school level and at college level.

Table 5.32

Patient's Suggestions for Improving Health Rights Information

Suggestions for Improving Health Rights Information	*Government Hospital*	*Private Hospital*	*Total Response**
Display on the main entry of hospital	46 (38.33)	49 (40.83)	95 (79.17)
Display on the OPD/Indoor Card	39 (32.5)	43 (35.83	82 (68.33)
Publicity by media	26 (21.67)	36 (30)	62 (51.67)
Health rights chapter to be included in text books	15 (12.5)	34 (28.33)	49 (40.83)

Figures in the bracket represent percentage.

* Multiple Responses.

Forms of Malpractice in the Hospitals

Malpractice is being done at different levels in providing health care to the patients. It varies at the level of doctors, pharmacists, diagnostic centres, etc.

When we asked our patients in government hospital regarding the source of their prescribed medicines, 29 (24.17%) replied that they bought the medicines from outside the hospital which otherwise they are supposed to have from the hospital. However, only 17 (14.17%) patients from private hospital get medicines inside the hospital. In private hospital, every patient has to buy the medicines from outside (see Table 5.33).

Table 5.33

Source of Procurement of Medicine

Source of Procurement of Medicine	*Government Hospital*	*Private Hospital*	*Total*
Within hospital	31 (25.83)	17 (14.17)	48 (40)
Outside hospital	29 (24.17)	43 (35.83)	72 (60)
Total	60 (50)	60 (50)	120 (100)

Figures in the bracket represent percentage.

Nearly forty-seven per cent of patients said that they paid money and got receipt for their treatment process, but 64 (53.33%) reported that they paid money but never received any kind of receipt for the payment made (see Table 5.34).

Table 5.34

Patient's Payment and Receiving Receipt for Treatment

Giving Payment and Receiving Receipt	*Government Hospital*	*Private Hospital*	*Total*
Yes	19 (15.83)	37 (30.83)	56 (46.67)
No	41 (34.17)	23 (19.17)	64 (53.33)
Total	60 (50)	60 (50)	120 (100)

After discussing the health rights of patients, we turn below to the ethics of doctors. Ethics will be discussed in terms of medical negligence, confidentiality and autonomy of doctors, etc. These are some of the issues which we will discuss in the following pages.

II

Medical Ethics among Doctors

Numerous indicators reflect a growing interest in ethical issues in medical and health care. Increasing media coverage includes discussion of ethical issues surrounding such developments as has been the case with reproductive technologies such as surrogate motherhood, cloning of human beings, etc. Moreover, professional organizations are devoting more time at their meetings and more space in their publications to discussion of ethical issues (Gottlieb et al., 1987). Against this background one might suspect an equivalent development of sociological interest in medical ethics. This is so because many issues in medical ethics are sociological topics of major interest. For example, work in the area of medical care ethics, particularly work focusing on the rights and duties of medical professionals and patients, bears directly on the evolving nature of the doctor-patient relationship (Stacey, 1985). Ethical analysis of medical and health care public policy has significant implication for such macro sociological issues as equality in access to care and the role of the professions in determining the availability of medical and health care services (Mechanic, 1979).

A review of recent medical sociology works reveals some coverage of an array of ethical issues in medical and health care (Mechanic, 1983; Susser et al., 1985; Mechanic and Aiken, 1986; Simmons and DiCanio, 1979). Much of this has focused on micro-ethical issues, such as the doctor-patient relationship and treatment decisions for critically ill patients (Crane, 1975). More recently there has been an extension to societal focused issues, such as the rationing of medical care (Mechanic, 1979). Lesser attention has been devoted to exploring ethical issues in the interactions between institutions and professionals to studying the dynamic relationships between the professions and society (Freidson, 1961). Some sociological attention also has been given to the rise and current interest in bioethics (Fox, 1974). The number of specific medical and health issues that have received ethical analysis is very large; they include such topics as death and dying, kidney dialysis, organ transplantation, clinical research, genetic counselling and screening, decision to extend or terminate life support system, allocation of scarce medical resources, cost containment, and ethical issues in the development of for-profit hospitals.

In India, not much work has been done on medical ethics; however, Desai (1988) tries to see the medical ethics in the continuity of indigenous and classical folk traditions. Wig (1985) discusses the forced population control measures as a medical and ethical issue. Desai and Chand (2007) lamented on the lacunae and absence of laws specifically with the duties of health facilities and personnel to provide medical treatment in emergency cases. Sriram et al. (1991) and Minocha (2010) have studied the discourse of informed consent in medical ethics along with field observation. There is not much work at the theoretical and empirical level which has been done on the medical ethics particularly in the Indian context.

Concept of Health

Before trying to understand heath rights and medical ethics, let us first begin by understanding what health means. *Health* is a very old term. In old English it was used as *haelen* (to heal), and in Middle English as *helthe,* meaning to be sound in body, mind, or spirit. The word was related to the practice of medicine. In ancient Greek civilization the definition of medicine was to 'prolong life and prevent disease' or, in other words, to keep people healthy. Similarly, medicine in ancient India was called Ayurveda, or the science of life or health. By the 17th century, the word 'restoration' began to be used in most medical textbooks. By the end of 19th century the word *health* was considered colloquial and was replaced with the word *hygiene,* which was considered more scientific (Cook, 2004).

First, the use of the word *state* in this definition is misleading. Health is dynamic and changes from time to time. For example, a person may be healthy in the morning; in the afternoon, he or she develops a headache and is thus not in the 'state' of health; in the evening, he or she may recover from the headache, thereby attaining the 'state' of the health again.

Table 5.35

Concept of Health as Viewed by the Doctors

Concept of Health	*Government Hospital*	*Private Hospital*	*Total Response**
Is energetic	9 (40.91)	6 (27.27)	15 (68.18)
Has good body build	8 (36.36)	5 (22.73)	13 (59.09)
Has good appetite	10 (45.45)	7 (31.82)	17 (77.27)
Has a good posture	11 (50)	5 (22.73)	16 (72.73)
Gets sound sleep	6 (27.27)	6 (27.27)	12 (54.54)
Able to work properly	9 (40.91)	5 (22.73)	14 (63.64)
Free from disease	12 (54.54)	7 (31.82)	19 (86.36)

Figures in the bracket represent percentage.

* Multiple Responses.

Like the patient, doctors have their concept of health which is based on their knowledge which they acquire during their study period and also during their practise of medical profession. We have tried to collect the views of doctors regarding their concept of health. Maximum number of doctors, i.e. 19 (86.36%) find good health in terms being from disease. A good number of doctors, i.e. 17 (77.27%) state that a good health is viewed in terms of good appetite. Another, 16 (72.73%) view good health in terms of good posture. Some doctors also view good health in terms of energy, good body build, and sound sleep and ability to work properly (see Table 5.35).

Regular Medical Check-up and Good Health

Nowadays medical fraternity and also the common people feel that keeping oneself healthy is one's own responsibility. People should not go to the hospital only when they suffer from some kind of disease, but they should periodically monitor their health. For monitoring their health, they should have periodic medical check-ups. In our study, doctors have emphasized on the importance of medical check-ups. Ninety-one per cent of the doctors feel that medical check-ups in advance are helpful in preventing disease. Another fifty per cent feel that for better cure advance medical check-ups are important. Equal number of doctors that is nearly forty-one per cent state that spending little in advance on medical check-ups and also advising others for advance check-up is always good for health. Some of them also mentioned that prevention is always better than cure.

Table 5.36

Why Regular Medical check-up is Necessary

Importance of Regular Health Check-up	*Government Hospital*	*Private Hospital*	*Total Response**
For healthy lifestyle	6 (27.27)	5 (22.73)	11 (50)
To prevent disease	12 (54.54)	8 (36.36)	20 (90.91)
To get well soon	5 (22.73)	2 (9.09)	7 (31.82)
To encourage others	6 (27.27)	3 (13.64)	9 (40.91)
Prevention is better than cure	3 (13.64)	2 (9.09)	5 (27.73)
Spending little on medical check-up keeps good health	5 (22.73)	4 (18.18)	9 (40.91)

Figures in the bracket represent percentage.

* Multiple Responses.

Further, we asked doctors to suggest some tips for living a healthy life. Doctors gave in multiple responses. Majority of the doctors, i.e. 18 (81.82%) mentioned about never ignoring your illness, meaning as and when you fall sick immediately report it to the doctor. Another sixteen doctors replied that regular check-ups are must to remain healthy. Another fifteen (68.18%) feel that eating of balanced diet is a must to remain healthy. Fourteen doctors opined that because of the sedentary lifestyle in the present society, physical exercise is must (see Table 5.37).

Table 5.37

Doctors' Perspective for Living Healthy Life

Suggestion for Healthy life	*Government Hospital*	*Private Hospital*	*Total Response**
Going for regular health check-up	9 (40.91)	7 (31.82)	16 (72.73)
Never ignore illness	11 (50)	7 (31.82)	18 (81.82)
Sleeping for at least 8–9 hours	7 (31.82)	6 (27.27)	13 (59.09)
Having a balanced diet	10 (45.45)	5 (22.73)	15 (68.18)
Having bath every day	6 (27.27)	3 (13.64)	9 (40.91)
Physical exercise	8 (36.36)	6 (27.27)	14 (63.64)

Figures in the bracket represent percentage.

* Multiple Responses.

Motivation to Choose Medical Profession

Every person, who joins a profession or enters into an occupation, is generally influenced by some motivating factors. These factors differ according to the nature of the occupation and also according to the particular socio-psychological background or circumstances of the incumbents. At the occupational level economic gain, security, high social prestige and power attached to the particular occupation may serve as important inducing factors for selecting a particular occupation. The medical profession, by its very nature as humanitarian and social service orientation, is looked upon by society with great respect. It provides economic gain and social prestige to the incumbents. To understand what types of factors are responsible for choosing the medical profession, the doctors in the present study are asked to give their opinion about the motivating factors for selection of medical profession. It is interesting to note that equal number of doctors, that is 17 (72.27%); motivated by service to mankind and respect they get in the society. However, 12 (54.54%) of them confess that medical profession gives them a chance to earn more money as compared to other professions. Nearly, forty-six per cent of the doctors are motivated by professional satisfaction in treating the patients (see Table 5.38).

Table 5.38

Motivation in Medical Profession

Motivation to choose Profession	*Government Hospital*	*Private Hospital*	*Total Response**
Service to human being	11 (50)	6 (27.27)	17 (77.27)
Earn more and more money	8 (36.36)	4 (18.18)	12 (54.54)
Professional satisfaction	6 (27.27)	4 (18.18)	10 (45.45)
Respect in society	11 (50)	6 (27.27)	17 (77.27)

Figures in the bracket represent percentage.

* Multiple Responses.

Doctor-Patient Relationship

The initial attitudes of doctors towards patients depict not only diagnosis and prognosis of the disease but also reflects doctor's feelings towards the patient as a professional, as a human being and as a service-oriented person.

Table 5.39

Doctor-Patient Relationship in Treatment Process

Relationship and Treatment process	*Government Hospital*	*Private Hospital*	*Total*
Yes	8 (36.36)	5 (22.73)	13 (59.09)
No	5 (22.73)	4 (18.18)	9 (40.91)
Total	13 (59.09)	9 (40.91)	22 (100)

Figures in the bracket represent percentage.

In our study, when we asked our respondents about the role of relationship between a doctor and a patient, it is interesting to note that nearly sixty per cent of the doctors feel that good relationship between the doctor and the patient helps in the treatment process (see Table 5.39).

Table 5.40

Contents of the Relationship between Doctor and Patient

Contents of the Relationship	*Government Hospital*	*Private Hospital*	*Total Response**
To clear doubts of patients regarding diseases	7 (53.85)	4 (30.77)	11 (84.61)
Both find themselves familiar	3 (23.08)	3 (23.08)	6 (46.5)
Social responsibility	5 (38.46)	4 (30.77)	9 (69.23)
Patients' mind is diverted from tensions	4 (30.77)	1 (7.69)	5 (38.46)
Professional ethics	3 (23.08)	2 (15.38)	5 (38.46)

Figures in the bracket represent percentage.

* Multiple Responses.

Further, regarding the content of the relationship between doctors and patients, nearly eighty-five per cent of the doctors mention that while interacting with the patient, they want to clear the doubts of patients in terms of the disease and the process of treatment. Ultimately the clarity of doubts helps in the treatment process. Around 9 (69.23%) doctors view that social interaction with the patient is their social responsibility. Five of them feel that by having social interaction with the patient, the mental tension is diverted and also helps in acting according to professional ethics (see Table 5.40).

Table 5.41

Behaviour of Doctors with the Patients

Behaviours of Doctors with Patients	*Government Hospital*	*Private Hospital*	*Total Response**
Cooperative	6 (27.27)	5 (22.73)	11 (50)
Normal	11 (50)	2 (9.09)	13 (59.09)
Emotional	1 (4.54)	2 (9.09)	3 (13.64)
Friendly	2 (9.09)	3 (13.64)	5 (22.73)

Figures in the bracket represent percentage.

* Multiple Responses.

Table 5.41 provides the behaviour of the doctors with the patients. Nearly sixty per cent of the doctors maintain that they have normal behaviour with their patients, whereas fifty per cent of the doctors told that they are cooperative with their patients.

Five (22.73%) are friendly with their patients and another 3 (13.64%) are emotive with their patients.

Doctors and their Medical Oath

Table 5.42 shows the doctors' remembrance of the oath taken by them after completing their medical course. Almost sixty-eight per cent of the doctors mention that they know the name of the oath taken by them, whereas nearly thirty per cent do not remember the name of the oath taken by them. This shows that almost one-third of the doctor, do not even bother to remember the name of the oath. Further, we asked our respondents to tell the contents of the oath, seventy per cent of them replied in bits and pieces.

Table 5.42

Knowing the Name of the Oath taken by Doctors

Know the Name of the Oath	*Government Hospital*	*Private Hospital*	*Total*
Yes	11 (50)	4 (18.18)	15 (68.18)
No	2 (9.09)	5 (22.73)	7 (31.82)
Total	13 (59.09)	9 (40.91)	22 (100)

Figures in the bracket represent percentage.

Medical Ethics and Doctors

Medical ethics are not merely a moral code but a legally sanctioned code of conduct acceptable and normal within the medical profession. This does not mean that morality or moral theories do not influence medical ethics, but medical ethics must be understood, analysed and practised from a rational standpoint. This rational component of professional conduct is legally codified under the code of medical ethics of the legally constituted medical council with which all qualified medical practitioners must be registered.

The registrations as well as the conduct as per the code of ethics are essential because, 'doctors use technical skills and expertise which the untrained person does not possess. Possessing these skills gives him great power over his patients who by the very fact of being patients are dependent, ill and vulnerable. In caring for his patients, a doctor makes a series of judgments and decisions which, patients have the right to expect, are made fairly in the light of the doctor's knowledge and experience' (British Medical Association, 1986). Thus, although the code of medical ethics is for the self-regulation of the profession, it is there in order to fulfil certain rights and expectations of the patient. In a nutshell, the code describes the doctor's duties towards the patient. If these rights are not fulfilled or duties are not performed, then the doctor in question loses his or her right to be part of the profession.

The Medical Council of India under its Medical Council Act, 1956 has recently, i.e. in 2002 made the regulations relating to the professional Conduct, Etiquette and Ethics for registered medical practitioners.

Table 5.43

Doctors and Ethical Elements in their Profession

Doctors and Ethical Elements in their Profession	*Government Hospital*	*Private Hospital*	*Total Response**
Respect for autonomy	11 (50)	5 (22.73)	16 (72.73)
Beneficence and Non-malfeasance	9 (40.91)	3 (13.64)	12 (54.54)
Justice	7 (31.82)	2 (9.09)	9 (40.91)
Informed consent	10 (45.45)	5 (22.73)	15 (68.18)
Truthfulness and confidentiality	5 (22.73)	2 (9.09)	7 (31.82)

Figures in the bracket represent percentage.

* Multiple Responses.

There are five major elements of ethics in the medical profession. They are respect for autonomy of medical professionals, beneficence and non-malfeasance, justice to all patients, informed consent and truthfulness and confidentiality in the medical profession. We presented these above ethical elements to the doctors and asked them to provide their preferences in the order of priority for the medical ethics. Nearly seventy-three per cent of the doctors mentioned that autonomy of the doctor is most important in the medical profession. Another fifteen (68.18%) gave priority to informed consent in their profession. Around 12 (54.54%) doctors maintain that medical profession is basically a profession of beneficence and non-malfeasance. To provide justice to all irrespective of their strata is another element of ethic in the medical profession (see Table 5.43).

Professional Ethics and Treatment to Patient

Professional ethics of a doctor suggest that a doctor is supposed to treat the patient irrespective of caste, class, ethnic, gender and other biasness. We simply asked our respondents if they can refuse treatment to the patient. As many as 9 (40.91%) doctors straight way replied that they can refuse treatment whereas majority of the doctors, i.e. 59.09 per cent still maintain that they cannot refuse treatment to any patient (see Table 5.44).

Table 5.44

Can a Doctor Refuse Treatment?

Can a doctor Refuse Treatment?	*Government Hospital*	*Private Hospital*	*Total*
Yes	6 (27.27)	3 (13.64)	9 (40.91)
No	7 (31.82)	6 (27.27)	13 (59.09)
Total	13 (59.09)	9 (40.91)	22 (100)

Figures in the bracket represent percentage.

Table 5.45

Reasons for Refusing Treatment

Reason for Refusing Treatment	*Government Hospital*	*Private Hospital*	*Total Response**
If the doctor himself is not well	3 (33.33)	2 (22.22)	5 (55.55)
If he has had a bad experience in the past	4 (44.44)	3 (33.33)	7 (77.78)
In odd hours	1 (11.11)	2 (22.22)	3 (33.33)
There is no legal obligation to treat a patient after duty hours	5 (55.55)	3 (33.33)	8 (88.89)
Doctor treats a patient in emergency on ethical grounds	6 (66.67)	1 (11.11)	7 (77.78)
Due to non-availability of certain facilities, instruments, medicines, staff, etc.	4 (44.44)	3 (33.33)	7 (77.78)
Already busy with other patients	3 (33.33)	1 (11.11)	4 (44.44)

Figures in the bracket represent percentage.

* Multiple Responses.

The doctors who refuse to treat the patient have shared their reasons for it. We received responses in the multiple forms. Nearly eighty-nine per cent of the doctors say that there is no legal binding on them to treat a patient after their duty hours. Furthermore, seventy per cent of the doctors share that they treat a patient only when they think that it is an emergency; sometimes they had some bad past experience of treating a patient after their duty hours; they also refuse to treat a patient when there are no facilities available to treat the patients. Sometimes, doctors also refuse to treat the patient, if they are already occupied with the treatment process of other patient or if they themselves are not well. Some doctors also refuse to treat patient in odd hours (see Table 5.45).

Table 5.46 shows the doctors' immediate response towards the person who is sick or injured outside the hospital. Fifty per cent of the doctors mention diplomatically that it depends upon the situation of the person. However, nearly forty-six per cent of the doctors replied that they will immediately provide first aid to the patient irrespective of any situation. And 8 (36.36%) doctors mentioned that they will immediately inform their relatives.

Table 5.46

Response of Doctor Towards Sick or Injured Outside the Hospital

Response	*Government Hospital*	*Private Hospital*	*Total Response**
To provide him/her first Aid	7 (31.82)	3 (13.64)	10 (45.45)
To admit him/her in nearby health centre	3 (13.64)	2 (9.09)	5 (22.73)
To inform his/her relative	5 (22.73)	3 (13.64)	8 (36.36)
Depends on situation	7 (31.82)	4 (18.18)	11 (50)

Figures in the bracket represent percentage.

* Multiple Responses.

Nature of Medical Ethics

Public health includes such a wide array of activities that only a culture of cooperation can bring all the agencies involved to work is consonance to obtain optimal results in terms of the health of the population. Quality of patient care also requires cooperation between doctors taking care at different times or across different specialties, and between doctors, nurses, etc. as well as relatives and friends attending to patients. Practitioners of different system of medicine need to cooperate to give the best of their system to individual patients as well as develop systems of integrated health care, that is, evolve a systematic approach to combine practices of the various knowledge systems so as to give maximum benefit to the patient and community (Tavistock Group, 1999).

Borrowing from feminist discourse and social psychology (Gilligan, 1982) this provides the notion of moving away from the ideal of a clinician who 'objectively' keeps his distance from the patient, who must not get emotionally concerned. In addition, it requires involving patients in decisions about their treatment and fulfilling subjective 'felt needs' to achieve patient satisfaction. Similarly, the community must be involved in deciding its health activities. Those viewed as the main 'beneficiaries' or the health services are to get both autonomy and justice, and therefore, their voices must be acknowledged as valid critical.

Table 5.47

Nature of Medical Ethics

Nature of Medical Ethics	*Government Hospital*	*Private Hospital*	*Total Response**
Doctor should always use 'medical power' for patient's benefit	11 (50)	5 (22.73)	16 (72.73)
Profession with conscience and dignity	12 (54.54)	6 (27.27)	18 (81.82)
Humanity or to save mankind	8 (36.36)	4 (18.18)	12 (54.54)
Respect and gratitude	7 (31.81)	3 (13.64)	10 (45.45)
Maintaining good medical practice	8 (36.36)	3 (13.64)	11 (50)
The health and life of my patient will be my first consideration	9 (40.91)	5 (22.73)	14 (63.64)
Do not use medical knowledge contrary to the laws of humanity	8 (36.36)	3 (13.64)	11 (50)
Respect the secrets which are confided to me	11 (50)	4 (18.18)	15 (68.18)

Figures in the bracket represent percentage.

* Multiple Responses.

We asked doctors very pertinent question about what includes medical ethics. The responses collected from the doctors are varied. Fifteen (68.18%) doctors maintained that they respect the confidentiality of the patient in terms of disease as well as about treatment. Nearly sixty-four per cent of the doctors view medical ethics in terms of health and life of patient as the prime concern. Exactly fifty per cent of the doctors feel that it is unfair to use medical knowledge contrary to the laws of humanity. As much as 16 (72.73%) feel that doctors should use their medical power and knowledge for the benefit of the patient. Majority of the doctors, i.e. 81.82 per cent maintain that medical profession is the profession of conscience and dignity (see Table 5.47).

Medical Negligence

Before discussing medical negligence, it would be important to understand the concept of negligence as such. Negligence may be defined as the 'breach of a duty caused by the omission to do something which a reasonable man, guided by those considerations which ordinarily regulate the conduct of human affairs would do, or doing something which a prudent and reasonable man would not do'. A shorter definition is that 'negligence as a tort is the breach of legal duty to take care which results in damage, undesired by the defendant to the plaintiff'. The definition involves three constituents of negligence: (1) A legal duty to exercise the due care on the part of the party complained of towards the party complaining the former's conduct within the scope of the duty; (2) breach of the said duty; (3) consequential damage.

For a doctor negligence means failure to act in accordance with the standards of reasonably competent medical men at the time. That is a perfectly accurate statement, as long as it is remembered that there may be one or more perfectly proper standards; and if a medical man conforms to one of those proper standards then he is not negligent. A doctor is not guilty of negligence if he has acted in accordance with a practice accepted as proper by a responsible body of medical men skilled in that particular art. Putting it the other way round, a doctor is not negligent, if he is acting in accordance with such a practice, merely because there is a body of opinion that takes a contrary view. At the same time, that does not mean that a medical man can obstinately and pig-headedly carry on with some old technique if it has been proved to be contrary to what is really substantially the whole of informed medical opinion.

As many as 436 people died last year due to Serious Adverse Events (SAE) during clinical trials. Investigations are now on to ascertain how many of the deaths were caused by drugs administered to the trial subjects. In 2011, 438 cases of SAE were reported, of which 16 were found to be due to clinical trials. The previous year, 668 cases of SAE were reported, of which 22 were caused due to trials. The union health ministry says there were alleged irregularities in nine cases of clinical trials during the last three years. Sources said that most of the clinical trials involving patients who died 'due to clinical trial' involved global pharmaceutical giants testing drugs for different types of cancer and antibiotics. The Supreme Court had recently pulled up the Centre for its insensitivity to scores of deaths and serious adverse effects to thousands during clinical trial of new drugs. 'We have taken steps like mandatory registration of clinical trial in ICMR registry to ensure that safety, rights and well-being of clinical trial subjects are protected,' said the health minister. The Health Ministry data shows the number of trials being approved has also gone down: from 529 permissions granted in 2010 to 283 in 2011 and 253 in 2012 (*The Times of India*, 2013A).

Lured by freebies and kickbacks from stent manufacturers, an increasing number of doctors are using the device even on heart patients who do not need them. So blatant has this practice become that in Hyderabad, eminent cardiologist Dr D. Seshagiri Rao, head, department of cardiology, Nizam's Insititute of Medicine (NIMS), was caught red-handed while accepting a bribe of ₹ 1.6 lakh from a stent supplier. He was arrested. Stents, the scaffolding devices inserted into blood vessels to keep them open, are used if the patient has more than 70 per cent block of an artery. But doctors confide that stents are used even when the block is less than 30 per cent. This not only inflates the bill, but increases the risk of a heart attack, say cardiologists. In fact, a study by National Heart and Lung Institute in the US found that 1–2 per cent of people who have stented arteries develop a blood clot at the stent site which can cause a heart attack or stroke.

'When stenting was introduced, it was hailed as a medical breakthrough, but patients are now being advised to go through the procedure even when the clot can be treated through aggressive medical intervention or through a bypass', says Dr B. Soma Raju, chairman of CARE Hospitals, Hyderabad, and a pioneer in this treatment. Dr Sai Satish, an international cardiologist at Apollo Hospitals, calls the trend 'criminal'. 'Last year I received at least four patients who were advised to go in for angioplasty when the problem could have been remedied through medication. We need a system to check this,' he says (*The Times of India*, 2013B).

As many as 2,644 people, called subjects, died during the clinical trials of 475 new drugs on human beings in last seven years and only 17 of the medicines were approved for marketing in India, the Centre has informed the Supreme Court. Union health and family welfare ministry said of the 57,303 enrolled subjects, 39,022 completed the clinical trials. 'Serious adverse events of deaths during the clinical trials during the mention period were 2,644, out of which 80 deaths were found to be attributable to the clinical trials (*The Times of India*, 2013C).

We asked doctors to give their views regarding medical negligence. Out of twenty-two doctors, almost one-third of the doctors admit that, there are cases of medical negligence in the medical facilities. However, 15 (68.18%) have totally refused that there are cases of medical negligence in the hospital. Contrary, to this in the private hospital setting, doctors are not ready to accept that they have the cases of medical negligence that is why only 2 (9.09%) doctors admitted that they do have cases of medical negligence (see Table 5.48).

Table 5.48

Incidence of Medical Negligence Reported by Doctors

Level of Education of Doctors	*Government Hospital*		*Private Hospital*	
	Yes, Incidence of Medical Negligence	*No Incidence of Medical Negligence*	*Yes, Incidence of Medical Negligence*	*No Incidence of Medical Negligence*
BDS	—	2 (9.09)	—	—
BAMS	—	—	1 (4.54)	4 (18.18)
MBBS	2 (9.09)	5 (22.73)	—	—
MD/MS	3 (13.64)	1 (4.54)	1 (4.54)	3 (13.64)
Total	5 (22.73)	8 (36.36)	2 (9.09)	7 (31.82)

Figures in the bracket represent percentage.

* Multiple Responses.

To ascertain doctors' information regarding the forms of medical negligence, 19 (86.36%) mentioned that taking out of patients' organs without his/her consent is the most severe form of medical negligence. Nearly seventy-three per cent report that delay in treatment of the patient is also a form of medical negligence. Fifteen (68.18%) feel that wrong treatment is also medical negligence. Overdose of medicine is another form of medical negligence which has been mentioned by 14 (63.64%) (see Table 5.49).

Table 5.49

Forms of Medical Negligence

Forms of Medical Negligence	*Government Hospital*	*Private Hospital*	*Total Response**
Wrong treatment	10 (45.45)	5 (22.73)	15 (68.18)
Delay in treatment	12 (54.54)	4 (18.18)	16 (72.73)
Taking out patient's organs without his/her consent	12 (54.54)	7 (31.82)	19 (86.36)
Overdoses of medicine	9 (40.91)	5 (22.73)	14 (63.64)

Figures in the bracket represent percentage.

* Multiple Responses.

Out of the doctors who report that there are cases of medical negligence in the medical facility, sixty per cent opine that many times new drugs are given to patients on trial basis. This may be due to kick backs from the pharmaceutical companies or may be from the medical representative of the company who are visiting the doctors for the promotion of their medicines. Another 11 (73.33%) doctors feel that there is rampant use of medical devices like stent, etc. which are in reality not needed to the patients (see Table 5.50). Thus, the medical negligence is viewed in terms of drug administration to patients and also unnecessary use of medical devices which are not really needed by the patients.

Table 5.50

Nature of Medical Negligence

Nature of Medical Negligence	*Government Hospital*	*Private Hospital*	*Total Response**
New drug given to patient for trial	6 (40)	3 (20)	9 (60)
Use of devices like stent, etc. not needed to patients	6 (40)	5 (33.33)	11 (73.33)

Figures in the bracket represent percentage.

* Multiple Responses.

Table 5.51
Causes of Doctors' Medical Negligence

Causes of Medical Negligence	*Government Hospital*	*Private Hospital*	*Total Response**
Do not scrutinize the patients properly	4 (54.14)	1 (14.28)	5 (71.43)
Busy schedule	1 (14.28)	2 (28.57)	3 (42.86)
No proper consultation with other senior doctors about the illness	1 (14.28)	—	1 (14.28)
Due to apathy between doctor and patient	4 (54.14)	2 (28.57)	6 (85.71)
Economic consideration	4 (54.14)	2 (28.57)	6 (85.71)

Figures in the bracket represent percentage.

* Multiple Responses.

It is equally important to look into the causes of medical negligence at doctors' level. When we tried to gather information about the causes of medical negligence from the patient, we received several responses. We tried to sort out some of the common responses. Doctors think that due to apathy of doctors to serve the patients or loss of feeling for mankind and economic considerations are most important causes of medical negligence. Almost seventy per cent of the doctors state that before treatment, doctors do not scrutinize patients' medical history, etc. Some doctors feel that overburdened doctors and avoidance of consultation with other doctors also pushes them towards incidences of medical negligence.

Doctors and Information to Patients

The manifestations of people's aggression can be seen in the sharp increase in the number of strikes by physicians all over the country, a steady and rapid decline of medical ethics, the flourishing of corrupt practices, the exaction of capitation fees by medical colleges, and rising commercialization in the medical profession. Indeed, doctors are no longer ashamed of negligence but take it as part of their 'professional hazard'. This was shown by the Lentin Commission report on the J.J. Hospital drug deaths in Mumbai. Undoubtedly, the medical profession requires a fresh approach with the patient as the focus of all attention. A crucial aspect of this, hitherto neglected, is the patients' right to information. The average patient relies completely on health professionals as if they can work miracles. The medical world does not feel morally responsible about informing the patient that a substitute and potentially less harmful medicine is available, though it may not produce the same quick results. Giving complete information to the patient is also necessary. For instance, it is common for patients to stop medication the moment they feel they are 'cured'. This is especially true of an antibiotic which yields its benefits only when the full course is taken (*The Times of India*, 1990).

Doctors are keen to reply about the medical information they share with their patients. The information which they share with their patient ranges from medicine to the side-effects of medicine and how to take medicine. Maximum number of doctors, i.e. 19 (86.36%), always tell their patients about the side-effects of medicine, whereas 15 (68.18%) doctors tell their patient about the full course of antibiotics. They tell their patients that if you will not take the full course of treatment your disease might recur shortly. Fourteen doctors said that they never forget to tell their patients about not stopping medicinal course even if they are cured. Doctors think that generally patients stop taking prescribed medicines by as soon as they feel that they are cured. Nearly 13 (59.09%) doctors tell their patients about the substitute of medicines because sometimes a particular brand of medicine is not available (see Table 5.52).

Table 5.52

Information Given to the Patient by Doctors

Information to Patient	*Government Hospital*	*Private Hospital*	*Total Response**
Do not stop medication till the doctor's advice	9 (40.91)	5 (22.73)	14 (63.64)
Full course of antibiotics is must	11 (50)	4 (18.18)	15 (68.18)
Tell them about substitute of medicine	9 (40.91)	4 (18.18)	13 (59.09)
Tell them about side-effects of medicine	12 (54.54)	7 (31.82)	19 (86.36)

Figures in the bracket represent percentage.

* Multiple Responses.

Informed Consent

We came to know from our doctors about the informed consent and type of treatment. Majority 19 (86.36%), of doctors replied that in surgical treatment, informed consent is a must, 16 (72.73%) replied in favour of organ transplant and 12 (54.54%) doctors have replied that even in normal treatment, informed consent is necessary.

Table 5.53

Informed Consent and Type of Treatment

Type of Treatment	*Government Hospital*	*Private Hospital*	*Total Response**
Surgical treatment	11 (50)	8 (36.36)	19 (86.36)
Organ Transplant	11 (50)	5 (22.73)	16 (72.73)
Normal treatment	8 (36.36)	4 (18.18)	12 (54.54)

Figures in the bracket represent percentage.

We asked our doctors regarding the informed consent. Around 12 (54.54%) doctors straight way replied that informed consent is a must, even in case of emergency medical care. However, 10 (45.45%) feel that there is no need to ask the patient for the medical care as it is more important to treat the patient (see Table 5.54).

Table 5.54

Can the Emergency Treatment be given without Consent?

Can Emergency treatment be given to the Patient?	*Government Hospital*	*Private Hospital*	*Total*
Yes	8 (36.36)	4 (18.18)	12 (54.54)
No	5 (22.73)	5 (22.73)	10 (45.45)
Total	13 (59.09)	9 (40.91)	22 (100)

Figures in the bracket represent percentage.

Regarding the obstacles in the taking the consent from the patient, doctors' responses are received in the multiple form. As many as 83.33 per cent of the doctors feel that it is very difficult to explain the technicality of the treatment to the patients as majority of the patients are either illiterate or they do not have any knowledge of treatment. Similarly, seventy-five per cent of the doctors' opinion is that it is very difficult for them to explain the line of treatment as the language becomes the barrier. Nearly, sixty per cent of the doctors mentioned that non-availability of relatives/guardian at the time of treatment, patients' inability to talk to doctor and at the same time non-availability of guardian/relatives and absence of other methods to inform to the patient for the treatment (see Table 5.55).

Table 5.55

Obstacles in taking the Consent of the Patients

Obstacles in Obtaining Consent	*Government Hospital*	*Private Hospital*	*Total Response**
It is not possible to communicate the relevant information to the patient because of a language barrier	5 (41.67)	4 (33.33)	9 (75)
Steps have been taken to find means of communicating but no such means have been found	5 (41.67)	2 (16.67)	7 (58.33)
Patient are unable to understand the technicality of treatment	7 (58.33)	3 (25)	10 (83.33)
In case of emergency, patients' inability to talk to doctor	4 (33.33)	3 (25)	7 (58.33)
Patients' guardian/parents are not with the patient	5 (41.67)	2 (16.67)	7 (58.33)

Figures in the bracket represent percentage.

* Multiple Responses.

Table 5.56

Format of Consent

Format of Consent	*Government Hospital*	*Private Hospital*	*Total Response**
Consent must be related to treatment	11 (50)	6 (27.27)	17 (77.27)
Consent must be informed	9 (40.91)	6 (27.27)	15 (68.18)
Consent must be voluntary	4 (18.18)	2 (9.09)	6 (27.27)
Consent must not be obtained through fraud or misrepresentation	9 (40.91)	3 (13.64)	12 (54.54)

Figures in the bracket represent percentage.

* Multiple Responses.

Regarding the format of the consent for the treatment, 17 (77.27%) of the doctors replied that the consent must be related only to that particular treatment of the diseases which a particular person is going for. Another 15 (68.18%) opined that whatever consent the patient gives, it should be communicated to the doctor. The view that there should be no pressure on the patient for giving consent for the treatment is shared by nearly twenty-eight per cent of the doctors. Around 12 (54.54%) doctors strongly believe that consent must not be obtained through fraudulent means or misrepresentation of facts (see Table 5.56).

Confidentiality of Patient

Keeping confidentiality of the patient is another attribute of medical ethics of doctors. Table 5.57 provides information regarding doctors' views on the confidential information of the patients in terms of their disease and treatment. Exactly fifty per cent of the doctors mentioned that they keep their patients' information as confidential, whereas 22.73 per cent of the doctors maintain that it depends upon the situation. Only 6 (27.27%) maintain that they do not bother to keep confidentiality of the disease and treatment process of their patients.

Table 5.57

Confidential Information of Patient's Disease and Treatment

Keeping Information of Patient Confidential	*Government Hospital*	*Private Hospital*	*Total*
Yes	9 (40.91)	2 (9.09)	11 (50)
No	2 (9.09)	4 (18.18)	6 (27.27)
Vary according to situation	2 (9.09)	3 (13.64)	5 (22.73)
Total	13 (59.09)	9 (40.91)	22 (100)

Figures in the bracket represent percentage.

Doctors and Better Health Care

How can the doctor contribute in making the lives of people better other than treatment? Multiple responses have been received while tabulating and classifying the answers of doctors. Majority of the doctors, i.e. seventy-three per cent of the doctor mentioned that giving guidelines for the prevention of disease is the best method for better health. Similarly, another 14 (63.64%) of the doctors feel that regular medical check-ups and following a healthy lifestyle can make people healthy. There should be minimum charges for consulting doctors, cracking down on health care fraud, providing free preventing care, and urgent treatment of health care were also mentioned (see Table 5.58).

Table 5.58

Doctors Efforts for Better Health Care

Doctors Efforts for better Health Care	*Government Hospital*	*Private Hospital*	*Total Response**
Urgent treatment of health problem	8 (36.36)	5 (22.73)	13 (59.09)
Improving health care quality and efficiency	9 (40.91)	7 (31.82)	16 (72.73)
Providing free preventive care	3 (13.64)	—	3 (13.64)
Preventing disease and illness	10 (45.45)	6 (27.27)	16 (72.73)
Cracking down on health care fraud	8 (36.36)	—	8 (36.36)
Instructions for healthy lifestyle	7 (31.82)	7 (31.82)	14 (63.64)
Regular medical check-up	9 (40.91)	5 (22.73)	14 (63.64)
Minimum charges for treatment	6 (27.27)	5 (22.73)	11 (50)

Figures in the bracket represent percentage.

* Multiple Responses.

Doctors and Health Rights of Patients

The medical profession is considered a noble profession because it helps in preserving life. We believe life is God-given. Thus, a doctor figures in the scheme of God as he stands to carry out His command. A patient generally approaches a doctor/hospital based on his/its reputation. Expectations of a patient are twofold: doctors and hospitals are expected to provide medical treatment with all the knowledge and skill at their command and secondly they will not do anything to harm the patient in any manner under any circumstances. Though a doctor may not be in a position to save his patient's life at all times, he is expected to use his special knowledge and skill in a most appropriate manner keeping in mind the interest of the patient who has entrusted his life to him. Therefore, it is expected that a doctor carries out necessary investigation or seeks a report from the patient. Further, unless it is an emergency, he obtains informed consent of the patient before proceeding with any major treatment, surgical operation, or even invasive investigation. Failure of a doctor and hospital to discharge this obligation is essentially a tortious liability. A tort is a civil wrong (*right in rem*) as against a contractual obligation (*right in personam*) – a breach that attracts judicial intervention by way of awarding damages. Thus, a patient's right to receive medical attention from doctors and hospitals is essentially a civil right. The relationship takes the shape of a contract to some extent because of informed consent, payment of fee, and performance of surgery/providing treatment, etc. while retaining essential elements of tort.

The Constitution of India does not provide any special rights to the patient. In fact, the patients' rights are basically indirect rights, which arise or flow from the obligations of a physician or health care provider under the Indian Medical Council (Professional Conduct, Etiquette and Ethics) Regulations, 2002. However, the basic rights of a patient, such as the right to know about his condition, or the right to participate in treatment decision-making do not exist in reality in medical practice. If at all, they exist only on paper or in philosophical talks and discourses. People have an expectation that if anything wrong occurs or is done by medical professionals, then justice should invariably be done. It is reasonable for a patient to expect medical doctors to take into consideration all relevant factors involved in the treatment. At the same time, it is reasonable for the medical professional to provide all reliable technical or non-technical information about the treatment/surgery in one go to the patient. However, decision-making still remains in the hands of health care professionals.

The basic principle is that medical doctors and associated medical professionals are responsible and liable for wrongs and failures in the performance of their medical duties towards patients. In India, generally Section 304–A of the Indian Penal Code (IPC), 1860 is the relevant provision under which a complaint against a medical practitioner for alleged criminal medical negligence is registered. Section 337 of the IPC deals with hurt caused by an act endangering life or personal safety of others. Section 338 of the IPC relates to grievous hurt by an act endangering life and personal liberty of others. However, the simple lack of care attracts only civil liability. Therefore, only civil negligence may not be enough to hold a medical professional criminally liable (Nayak, 2004).

Practice and understanding of health rights can only be understood when we understand the views of users of health care as well as from the providers of health care. In our study maximum number of doctors, i.e. 19 (86.36%) feel that free choice of health services is the most important aspect of health right. As many as 18 (81.82%) doctors feel that the patients right is to get equal treatment irrespective of one's caste, class, ethnic, economic background and occupational background. To receive adequate health care is the right of the patients has been mentioned by nearly seventy per cent of the doctors. There are many emergency situations where patient needs immediate care without delay has been viewed by 63.64 per cent of the doctors. A large number of doctors also feel that patient should be treated with dignity and in the welfare state it is the duty of the government to provide health care to its citizen. Some of the doctors view that the right of patient is also in terms of getting the receipts of medicine, diagnostic tests and fee of doctors (see Table 5.59).

Table 5.59

Health Rights according to Doctors

Health Rights as Viewed by Doctors	*Government Hospital*	*Private Hospital*	*Total Response**
Live with dignity	8 (36.36)	6 (27.27)	14 (63.64)
Government's responsibility to provide health services	10 (45.45)	6 (27.27)	16 (72.73)
Fixed charges for health services	8 (36.36)	3 (13.64)	11 (50)
Receipts of medicine, diagnostic tests and of consultation fee of doctor	4 (18.18)	3 (13.64)	7 (31.82)
Free choice of health services	12 (54.54)	7 (31.82)	19 (86.36)
Confidentiality of patients' disease	12 (54.54)	5 (22.73)	17 (77.27)
Continuity of health care	10 (45.45)	5 (22.73)	15 (68.18)
Adequate health care	10 (45.45)	6 (27.27)	16 (72.73)
Well diagnosed treatment	4 (18.18)	4 (18.18)	8 (36.36)
Emergency treatment of disease like accidents, etc.	9 (40.91)	5 (22.73)	14 (63.64)
Equal treatment to all irrespective of patients caste, class, sex, age, etc.	10 (45.45)	8 (36.36)	18 (81.82)

Figures in the bracket represent percentage.

* Multiple Responses.

Doctors' Views about Organ Donation

Many doctors hope it will not only bring the spotlight on the poor rate of cadaver donation in the country, but also highlight the pathetic coordination between various states in this regard. It is, for instance, not easy for a solid organ such as the liver to be packed from Mumbai to Delhi or vice versa. Most states – except for Maharashtra, Tamil Nadu and Karnataka – do not even have a state-government-run organization to coordinate a cadaver donation programme. 'At present, there are no guidelines on who should be talking to whom. Doctors from private hospitals talk to their counterparts in other states and transfer organs, with ethics taking a backseat and monetary considerations as the only guiding light', said by a doctor.

A cadaveric donation occurs when the family of a patient who has been declared brain dead agrees to donate his or her organs (mainly kidneys and liver). But the numbers in most states except Tamil Nadu are extremely low. Mumbai, which was the first in the country to set up an official body, called the Zonal Transplantation Coordination Centre, to oversee cadaveric organ donations, registers less than 20 such donations a year. In 2004, an attempt to send a liver from Mumbai to Pune failed as no proper rules had been drawn up for the purpose. More recently, Chennai's heart transplant surgeon K. Cherian wrote to the Maharashtra Government complaining about hearts not being retrieved in Mumbai's hospitals. In contrast, the US, which is geographically much bigger than India, has a central organ bank that coordinates about patients who are to receive organs. The cadaver donation and organ transplant mechanism in India needs to be unshackled immediately from red tape. Too much of bureaucratization and arbitrariness are the twin problems that block life-saving transplants in most states in India. The Gujarat Government's move to help ailing Vilasrao Deshmukh is welcome; but this should be rule for everyone and not an exception for the privileged (*The Times of India*, 2012).

Table 5.60

Favour/Disfavour Organ Donation

Favouring/Disfavouring of Organ Donation by Doctors	*Government Hospital*	*Private Hospital*	*Total*
Yes	7 (31.81)	5 (22.72)	12 (54.54)
No	4 (18.18)	3 (13.64)	7 (31.81)
In some cases	2 (9.09)	1 (4.54)	3 (13.64)
Total	13 (59.09)	9 (40.91)	22 (100)

Figures in the bracket represent percentage.

Table 5.60 shows doctors' response towards organ donation. It has been a big issue for discourse from ethical point of view among the masses as well as among the medical professionals. Around 12 (54.54%) doctors totally favour organ donation. According to them, it can save the life of a person. However, 7 (31.81%) doctors are quite opposed to the idea of organ donation as they feel that it is unethical to take out the organ of one person and transplant it in another person. Furthermore, according to them it will also increase the unethical practices in the medical profession. Only 3 (13.64%) doctors maintained that donation of organ can be useful in some cases. Donation and transplantation of organ will depend upon the nature and situation of the patient and donor.

6

Violation of Medical Ethics and Health Rights of Patients

In the present chapter we will discuss some of the case histories on violation of medical ethics and health rights.

During the last two decades ethical issues in medicine are receiving greater attention. This applies to both medical practice as well as medical research. The advances in medicine, changing perceptions of the public and physicians, greater availability of information to the common man and political developments have all led to the ethical aspect of medicine becoming more relevant. Ethics are no more just a matter of special situation to be tackled by those working in frontier areas of medical practice and research.

Charak – the celebrated Indian physician of the bygone era said 'Health is vital for ethical, artistic, material and spiritual development of man'. According to Buddha, 'of all the gains, the gains of health are the highest and the best'. The overriding importance of good health to humankind is to be found in ancient literatures from other parts of the world as well.

Against this background, the lack of training to medical professionals on ethical aspects is well recognized. In India, the Indian Council of Medical Research (ICMR) has published a policy statement on ethical considerations involved in research on human subjects.

The all pervading ethos of the medical profession is to help the patient in the best possible way to get rid of the diseases. For a doctor, therefore, the patient is above everything else. Even if the deadliest enemy of the doctor makes an approach to him, the latter is obliged to help him in curing the diseases. Service to patient, therefore, is the ultimate ethics for a doctor. It is this ethic which keeps the practitioners of professions held together. Another binding force is to consider the professional members in the ties of kinship bonds. Normally, if the dictates of ethics are followed, a doctor would not charge any fee to examine the close relations of another doctor, anywhere, any time. Besides, there are certain other norms which keep the profession and its practitioners autonomous. For instance, if one is under the treatment of a particular doctor – the other would not intervene.

The Medical Council of India and the State Medical Council are the guardians of the rightful observation of the normative ethics of the profession. In fact, one of the objectives of the Medical Council of India is to monitor the profession at various levels. However, whenever such offences are committed, the office of the Council does not take any cognizance unless complaints are lodged to the council. However, the Medical Council of India has made sought amendment to the Medical Council Act, 1954 in the year 1974 by amending that any contravention of medical ethics is a cognizable offence. The Medical Council is also empowered to set up and to decide suitable punishment to the offenders. Thus, the observations of medical ethics laid down by the council have statutory strength.

Our interviews with the doctors show that in normal course of treatment they observe the general idiom of professional ethics. However, there are cases where one can find deviance from the ethics. For instances, it is expected of a doctor not to administer heavy doses to a patient which might result in side-effects. But to get more money they resort to heavy dose along with polytherapy. A patient who is a victim of such treatments in the long run finds his health shattered. This is obviously a violation of ethics.

Yet another ethic of a doctor is to take the patient into confidence. During the course of treatment, ethically the doctor should make it clear to the patient about the nature of his ailment. He should be told boldly that the consequences of ailment would be fatal or not. Ethically one is entitled to take the patient into confidence.

However, the ethics of medical profession should not come in conflict with the larger interest of the society. Take for instance, the case of vasectomy and medical termination of child. Both these operations have a wider connotation in the interest of the country. But any leakage of such operation has worst social consequences. Hypothetically, if after vasectomy the wife happens to conceive a child, she would be ridiculed by the society. In the same way if the secret about the medical termination is disclosed, it might brand the woman as one with bad character. Though, the operations are a reality but it is ethical obligation of the doctors to maintain secrecy. Similar is the case of leprosy and venereal diseases. When a patient approaches a doctor, he discloses everything to the doctor. If the doctor leaks out the personal secret, it is not only violation of the professional ethics but also a betrayal of the patient. Below, we will discuss the Ethics of Doctors in Section-I and Health Rights of Patients in Section II.

Such ethical norms, which we found in the field, are presented below.

I

The physicians have obligations beyond those of their own patients, a broader responsibility towards the health of the society. A physician's advocacy for his patient should not be exclusive but inclusive of social policies. Child sex ratios in Punjab and Haryana, especially with the adverse sex ratio at birth, point towards rampant practice of female foeticide (Premi, 2001). It clearly suggests the advancement in technology to know the health and sex of the foetus has turned out to be misused largely. People have started consulting the doctors not for the well-being of foetus in the womb but to know the sex of the foetus. On the other hand, doctors also readily tell them about the sex of the foetus because in return they get good amount of money. It is a big ethical issue. However, the state and central government have made it an offence to go for the amniocenteses test for knowing the sex of the foetus. One doctor reported:

Case I

One patient came to me for the amniocentesis test. I told her about the foetus that everything is all right. But she insisted me to tell the sex of the foetus. She also narrated her plight that she is already having four daughters and now she wants to have a son. Being a part of the same society, I listened to her sympathetically.

Though, as a doctor and according to medical ethics, I should not have told her about the sex of the foetus, but as she insisted, I had to tell her about it. Later on she got her abortion done.

For centuries now, mankind has tampered with the laws of nature and health care has provided him with some of the tools to do so. Nature's sex-ratio balance has been disturbed by the intervention of medical technology in terms of knowing the sex of foetus and then killing it if it is female. Therefore, it has also resulted into many social problems. A doctor dealing with this problem has an added responsibility to ensure that social balance is maintained.

Contrary to the popular perception, the government is designed to be competent machinery with detailed systems in place to avoid any crisis in treatment process. Drug stocks in public health system are meant to be regularly monitored and the suppliers should be kept in loop about future requirements. Hence, all drug stock-outs are created – either out of neglect or out of self-interest. No drug stock-out is ever an unanticipated one. Who then is responsible for these stock-outs? It is rarely an individual but usually a result of actions (or inactions) by a group or the entire system. A drug stock-out requires some negligence, compliance and efforts by all actors in the medical organization.

This points to several systemic weaknesses that are difficult but essential to address. There is a culture of neglect where the health establishment is geared for minimal action to disturb the status quo. There is also a deeply ingrained mindset of mutual protection. Despite a looming crisis, people within the system rarely raise an alarm. The matter only reaches a head when word gets out to the media or some senior calls for explanations. Until then the system protects itself, while poor patients wait for the health system to deliver.

We will put down certain newspaper reporting about negligence of doctors.

Case II

Acting on a *Tribune* report about refusal of treatment to a patient of burn injuries, who later died, the Haryana Health Department today found a government doctor guilty of negligence in discharging his duty and referred the matter to the higher authorities for disciplinary action against him.

The victim, X of Siwani town in Bhiwani district, was taken to the Civil Hospital on 24 May with around 80 per cent burn injuries. The doctor on emergency duty refused to admit her, asking the family to take her to Bhiwani since it was a police case and a medico-legal report (MLR) would be required. After waiting for around 40 minutes at Civil Hospital, the family took X to a private hospital. The Civil Hospital did not provide an ambulance to shift her to the private one. The woman succumbed to her injuries the next day. In a letter to the Additional Chief Secretary seeking disciplinary action, Dr Y, Director General (DG-Health Services), said the Civil Surgeon, Hisar, found the doctor negligent in discharging his duty. Citing a Supreme Court observation that stated that there is no legal impediment for a medical professional to attend to an injured person needing immediate medical assistance, the DG issued instructions to the Civil Surgeons for emergency treatment. 'There is no doubt that the effort to save the person should be the top priority not only of a medical professional, but even of the police or any other citizen who happens to be connected with the matter or who happens to notice such an incident', the apex court had stated. The DG said the Health Department had issued guidelines on 12 July 2013, regarding referring patients to higher centres.

Case III

A woman delivered a baby outside the General Hospital, after the authorities refused to perform her delivery. The woman, who belonged to a poor family from X village in Y district, is brought to the General Hospital for delivery. Ironically, the doctors, who are 'busy' in a mega health camp organized by some Minister, therefore did not have time to see this woman. While the woman was crying in labour pain, the doctors told her family to take her to another hospital as they do not have the facilities to assist a delivery. This happened at a time when, as per the authorities' claims, several specialists from Hisar, Delhi, Chandigarh and Panchkula were there to examine patients in the mega camp. The hapless family brought the woman out of the hospital and her husband rushed to fetch a rickshaw. However, the woman started delivering her baby while she was still within the four walls of the hospital complex, but outside the hospital building. She took the support of a scooter parked in the hospital and delivered her baby out in open.

Case IV

X, a female, who was visiting the civil hospital since the first month of her pregnancy in December 2012 for antenatal check-ups, complained about stoppage of growth of the foetus after 23 weeks. She said that despite complaints, the doctors at the gynaecology department found the pregnancy normal and offered no treatment for foetal growth. She told that even when she complained repeatedly about infection, allergies and severe stomach pain, no ultrasound was conducted, even though doctors observed that the foetus had not grown. She was instead sent to the skin department when she reported rashes after 33 weeks of pregnancy, without conducting any tests on her womb. Finding the doctors at the civil hospital negligent, she then approached Government Medical College and Hospital, where finally an ultrasound was conducted and it was found that the foetus had crimped. She then went to a private nursing home where she learnt that the government hospital had never brought to her knowledge that her baby was not growing in the uterus as even at 33 weeks the growth of the foetus growth was that of 26 weeks.

II

Following case histories are about the violation of health rights of the patients. Here these case histories will help us to analyse the issues of confidentiality, right to get equal health care, informed choice of treatment, medical negligence and confidentiality.

Case I

M is a 40-year-old man from the X town suffering from minor ailment for last several weeks. He works as an executive Engineer in Electricity Board and has monthly income of ₹ 60,000. During the conversation he told that the doctor took five minutes for diagnosis, and after the diagnosis he prescribed the medicine and told him to come after a week. This is his second visit, he said. After initial check-up, doctor and the patient exchanged the views on his field of work and current news and Indian polity for 10 minutes. On the question of patient's background, patient admits that the economic status and education makes a difference in every sphere of life. He said, they charged more from me but I cannot queue-up for the minor ailments.

Case II

R is a 35-year-old woman from X village. Her husband works in the fields and has monthly income of about ₹ 5,000. She is suffering from Jaundice and has been taking treatment for last one month. She has spent almost ₹ 3,500 on her diagnosis and treatment. She said that doctor does not know about my residential status and never asked about it and also did not suggest anything about precautions to be taken. The doctor only continued/changed some medicines. She said that private practitioners provide the best service. Of course they charge more, but that cannot be helped. It is not a grocery shop where you have a choice of not buying any commodity if he is charging extra.

Case III

This is a young woman of around 25 years of age and visits a private hospital where I was having conversation with one doctor, who is a child specialist and his wife also runs a diagnostic centre in same premises. This patient came here on the recommendation of another doctor's prescription. In this case the doctor neglected the main issues of patient's query and asked: 'is this first child? Yes, you should go for all tests and all are necessary and don't try to be smart to avoid these tests'. It is important to notice that doctor did not provide any suitable reason for doing the diagnostic tests.

Case IV

A 42-year-old female is having a problem of obesity for last one and a half years and had taken her first treatment from a private clinic. She said that in her village there is no medical facility due to which she had to come to Bhiwani. There are only private clinics at her native place and she is not sure about the competence and degree of the doctors. According to her, private treatment is expensive and hence she discontinued the treatment. She said that she has hardly taken the *angreji dawai* as it did not suit her body. She said that the doctor diagnosed her for 2–3 minutes, checked her sugar level, blood pressure report and then prescribed medicines and injections. She takes medicine daily but there is no relief. When she asked about the reasons from the doctor for her not getting relief, the doctor told her to continue the medicines for one or two days more. The doctor suggests her that if these medicines will not work then he will prescribe heavy dose.

Case V

A female aged 47 years is admitted in government hospital for last three days. She had a fracture in her hand and injury on upper part of the body. She was living on rent in a city with her family. She waited at the emergency ward for about 20–25 minutes. When the doctor came, her son told him that it is a Medico-Legal Case (MLC). Then the doctor checked her and told her to do an X-ray and ultrasound from a private lab which is located outside the hospital as hospital's X-ray and ultrasound machines are not working properly. They charged ₹ 480 for the report. She says that the doctor hardly visits the ward, usually; he visits either in the morning or in the evening. Her bedsheet has not been changed for last three days. She tells that there is biasness in their behaviour towards the patients in every aspect of examination. One who had good connections or had paid bribe, he/she gets better care. Nurses and even ward attendants also do not perform their duty; sometimes they consider themselves as powerful as doctors and rebuke the patients when they tell them of any problem.

Case VI

A male, 51 years old has been admitted to the government hospital for last eight days. He is being treated for fractured leg and hand. He got injured in a family dispute on the issue of land distribution. Though he was admitted by his son, but now he is alone here. He says that there is no proper care in the hospital and nurses are hardly present in the ward as they are busy with their personal work or gossips. There is no proper stand for drip and even his glucose bottle is tucked on the window. Nurses are not well experienced, and while giving injection, they cause great pain. He described – *'bhai ye nurse to is taryan sui lagvan san ki jani to bhans k sui lagavan sain, badi kattar han ye. Insaniyat naam ki koi chej nahi h yahan par'* (nurses give injection to him as if he is an animal and also they have shown no humanity). He is paying ₹ 100 per day, but not getting any receipt. Patient's meal is provided by the hospital authority. He described about the meal – *'Bhai un rotiyan n to kha k soch lek hasptal me dakhal rahna s'* (quality of food is very poor and it can make you fall sick).

Case VII

A 58-year-old male patient is admitted to the hospital for the treatment of anaemia. The patient tells that he is feeling weakness in his body and accompanied by numbness. His family members also said that he is looking very sick by his appearance. He came to the hospital with his son and the doctor admitted him. Two bottles of blood are given to him. When we asked him as to why he did not visit a government hospital, he replied that the government has opened up hospitals but there is no one to take care as well as no sufficient staff. His opinion regarding health right is: *'marij ka koi right nahi ji, balki marij ka kam hai marna'* (patients have no rights, because being sick means one has to die). Prescribed medicines are not available in the hospital's medical store and they have to buy these from outside. They are charged more than Maximum Price Rate (MRP) for these medicines. They sometimes match the prescribed medicine with the purchased medicine, but not always. The doctor writes medicines on a slip and medical store owner provides these medicines after seeing that slip. The medical store owner gives a bill on a rough paper but that is not a proper bill. A proper bill is provided only if the consumer insisted. In emergency situations, they say, it is important to get the medicines than to find faults. It is more important than money.

Case VIII

A 32-year-old male patient is brought to the hospital at 10 AM with stomach pain on right side. He is suffering for last two months. When he experienced pain for the first time, he took a pain killer. This relieved him of pain After that he went to a medical store and bought pain killers. He is taking pills as and when he feels pain without consulting any doctor. After persistent pain, he consults a doctor in a private hospital. His ultrasound report shows that he is suffering from Appendicitis. The doctor advises him for surgery. He takes the report and comes back home and consults another doctor, who advices him to go to another private doctor who would charge ten thousand rupees. After check-up, he is admitted for the Appendicitis operation. On the 2nd day after conducting relevant tests, he is taken to the operation theatre, operation was conducted. He was normal after the operation and discharged the next day with three days medicine course. But he again faces same problem on Sunday. He goes to the doctor and who prescribes him an injection. His brother got the injection from a medical store as per doctor's prescription, but nurse comes late and till then he suffered with pain. Patient is pointing to the carelessness of the ward staff and says that *'kuch to loha khota hai aur kuch lohar'* (Sometimes we turn a blind eye and sometimes they are not available when some injection or glucose is to be given).

Case IX

A 70-year-male patient is taken to the hospital at 8 AM with body pain and diarrhoea. At midnight he had suffered with loose motions and body pain. He is taken to the nearest private hospital at Charkhi Dadri, where he was given treatment. He paid ₹ 1,150 and was discharged immediately. He came back home, but did not get any relief, rather it got aggravated. Next morning he is again taken to a private hospital in Bhiwani, where he is treated for the illness and he got well. The patient explains that in every visit the doctor would spend about 3–4 minutes in investigation. The hospital was equipped with qualified staff and their fee charges were also nominal. He paid for the tests and medicines, but he did not ask for the bill and nor did they provide any bill for the paid amount. The patient says that doctor is equivalent to God *'Bhagwan aur Doctor ko kabhi naraaz mat karna, kyu ki Bhagwan naraaz to Aap Doctor k pass, aur Doctor naraaz tai Aap Bhagwan ke pass'* (Never annoy the God and the Doctor, because if you annoy the God, you will have to go to the doctor, and if you annoy the doctor, the God will call you).

Case X

A 78-year-old male patient is admitted to the hospital by his son and wife. He is having infection. After check-up and on the basis of report, doctor tells him that his lungs are totally damaged. He belongs to a poor family. His son is the only earning member, but now he is also in the hospital with him. There is no one to take care of him and his family. They cannot afford good treatment because of financial problem. Proper care is not given by the nurses and staff members because of his poor economic background. Doctor do not answer satisfactorily and make fun of him by saying that *'baba is umar me tera ghoda to ban nahi sakta'* (we cannot make you fit like a horse at this age). It reflects the apathy of doctors for the patient who has poor economic background.

Case XI

A 48-year-old female is admitted to a private hospital. Injections and medicines are given to her but she does not get any relief. She is taken to a government hospital. Doctor did not share with her anything about the disease. Finally it was the pharmacist who told her that she was suffering from cancer.

Case XII

Another 65-year-old male patient is admitted to a government hospital for lungs' problem. During last 7 days he had spent about ₹ 2,500. He is taking medicines for last 20 days, but without any relief. His body pain has increased. He is taken to the hospital in emergency ward by his son; the doctor has prescribed certain tests. After test they did not find the doctor to show his reports. After that the doctor asked them to arrange for two bottles of blood. Blood bank incharge asked him for bribe. He belongs to a BPL family; therefore he is not supposed to pay money. This was the patient's response about the hospital services – *bhai garib ki to har jagha mar hove* (since we are poor, therefore, nobody cares for us).

Case XIII

A 34-year-old female reports that she is a labourer and she is here in the government hospital for last eighteen days for her fractured leg. Before coming to the government hospital she was admitted in a private clinic for one day and they charged her one thousand rupees. When she did not feel any relief, then she came to the government General Hospital. Before the operation day the doctors asked her to pay ₹ 2,500 as the fee of anaesthesia doctor.

Case XIV

A 25-year-old female patient is taken to the hospital for child delivery. Delivery is held at Primary Health Centre. Due to negligence of the doctor water entered into the lungs of the newborn. She is referred to the General Hospital Bhiwani. She waited for admission in the emergency ward. Certain tests are prescribed which are to be done from outside the hospital. Doctor did not tell them about the illness of newborn. She did not ask the doctor about the condition of the newborn, as she feared that the doctor might get annoyed and stop treating the baby.

With regard to the qualitative analysis of case histories taken from the doctors and patients in terms of ethics and health rights, following conclusion is drawn:

Patients found that their socio-economic background does matter in getting the treatment, particularly in government hospital. In case of private hospital, they have to spend more money. Behaviour of doctors and nurses is very rude in the government hospital. They do not understand the pain and misery of the patient. However, few patients still regard the doctor as God. Few of them also reported that they have to pay more money for the services rendered, as there is no system of receipt. Receipt is only given, when they insist on it. Patients also feel that unnecessary diagnostic tests are done, which means they have to spend more money on tests. Doctors do not inform them about the need of the diagnostic tests. Doctors keep on changing medicines which means they do not have confidence on their treatment and consider a patient as their laboratory.

All the above instances are of patients who had come for treatment as indoor patients in government and private hospitals. It is clear that patients in government hospital complained of lack of infrastructure and facilities. The patients have to pay bribe to arrange for anaesthesia doctor and also arranging for blood. However, in the private hospital, they pay the charges, therefore, rooms and beds are better. Behaviour of the doctors and nurses are friendlier in private hospital as compared to government hospital.

There is a general complaint of patients in the government hospital about the dirty bedsheets, lack of proper stretcher, lack of proper stand for drips, etc. Only few patients get medicines in the government hospital, and in most cases they have to spend out of their pocket which sometimes forces them to shift to private hospital.

It is worth noting that the patients also find some nexus between prescription of medicines and the drugstore. The drugstore does not provide them with receipt. The delay in treatment also affects the recovery of the patient. Some of the patients feel that there is unnecessary delay in the treatment. It is more crucial in serious cases. People are willing to pay for private services because it saves their time, treatment starts immediately and doctors also listen to them. No patient has reported that they have an informed choice of the treatment.

7

Summary and Conclusion

The concept of right to health as a human right has recently emerged of ever-growing consciousness about the dignity of human life, all over the world. The right to health means that government must generate conditions in which everyone can be as healthy as possible. Such conditions range from ensuring availability of health services, healthy and safe working conditions, adequate housing and nutritious food.

Right to health and health care is a fundamental right under Article 21 of the Constitution of India. This Article of the Constitution casts a special obligation on the state to protect citizens' life from medical and other form of negligence. At the same time Article 21 of the International Covenant on Economic, Social and Cultural Right recognizes the 'right of every citizen to highest attainable standard of physical and mental health'.

There are some dominant theoretical paradigms for understanding a human right approach to health. Under utilitarianism, a right to health care should be justified if it contributes to the overall increase of net social utility. Communitarian theories of justice offer a relative account of justice and health care of public health, whereby the provision of health care is justified by the shared expression of values in a given community. Libertarian theories of justice take the principle of liberty as absolute and do not give to health any special standing. It supports national laws that guarantee negative freedom, but in general opposes the redistribution of resources required to fulfil positive rights. Egalitarian rights-based theory argues for a right to health care on the basis of 'equality of

Opportunity'. It proposes that social institutions affecting health care distribution should be arranged in such a manner so that each person in the society is able to have a fair share of normal range of opportunities.

The practice of medicine has a special place for ethics which is not so pronounced in other professions. Doctors are directly involved with the patient when he is in a most vulnerable position with the immediate issues of life and death, and of health and illness. To deal with this situation, doctors have certain personal and professional code of ethics that spell out certain limits for what constitutes acceptable and unacceptable behaviour. In the field of medicine, basic ethical conflicts are reflected in the struggle for control over knowledge, its use or misuse by professionals and the role of state in ensuring equity in health.

There are five main principles of health care ethics, namely, truthfulness and confidentiality, autonomy, informed consent, beneficence and non-maleficence and justice. The Kantian theory of ethics explains that whether the actions are right or wrong can be determined by reason, and the individual has a duty to act accordingly. Care-based theory of ethics is based on constructive ideas of mutual interdependence and emotional response. The ethics of care is a rejection of impartial, principle-driven, dispassionate reasoning and judgement that has often dominated the models and paradigms of bioethics. Communitarianism ethical theory drives from communal values, the common good, social goals, traditional practices and cooperative virtues. The major postulate of deontological theory of ethics is that we may not use or mistreat other people as a means to our happiness or that of others. Utilitarianism theory of ethics considers an action as morally right if its outcomes or consequences are good for the greatest number of population. It regards individual rights and considers the welfare of the people.

Number of sociological studies have researched on health care practices, doctor-patient communication, access to treatment and utilization of health care in public and private health facilities, preferences or choice of treatment, doctors as professionals, etc. Few studies have also been done on the cost of treatment, affordability and cost-benefit analysis. However, very few studies have been conducted on health rights and medical ethics. The review has been done to make an attempt to situate the ethics and health rights in the context of present study.

Health rights and medical ethics are related to one another. Health rights are exercised by people who use the health services, and medical ethics are reflected in the professional performance of doctors while delivering their health services. How the doctors' ethics are reflected in their medical profession and, in turn, how the health needs of patients are fulfilled is the task of the present study. Whether doctors treat the patients with dignity and pay value to their anxiety are the other dimensions to be explored in the study. Few case studies have also been taken to see the individual experience in context of health rights and medical ethics.

As the scope of medicine expands from clinical practice to mass interventions and realm of public health, ethical guidelines are very important for the code of conduct for physicians, the rights of patients and informed consent. Ethical analysis of medical health care has significant implication for issues like equality in access to care and role of medical profession in determining the availability of medical and health care services. Recently, the ethical guidelines provided by Indian Medical Council 'Regulation 2002' is aimed to improve the functioning of medical profession, as emerging concerns of organ transplantation, clinical trials, genetic manipulation, etc. has come into being. At the same time, health rights are also asserted by the patients who are more educated and with global exposure. Thus, it becomes relevant to understand the health rights and medical ethics in the context of doctors and users of health services, i.e. patients.

Thus, in our study we set out the following objectives:

Objectives of the Study

(i) To identify the socio-economic background of doctors and indoor patients.
(ii) To understand the meaning of health, health rights and medical ethics.
(iii) To comprehend the knowledge of the patients regarding their health rights.
(iv) To analyse the knowledge and practice of doctors regarding the medical ethics.
(v) To analyse the incidents of violation of health rights as experienced by the patients and doctors.

The purpose of our study is to understand the meaning of health, health rights and medical ethics. Therefore, hospital institutions are taken into account. Hospitals are comprised of doctors, patients and other paramedical staff. Out of the 21 districts, we randomly selected the Bhiwani district, which is one of the largest districts in the state of Haryana. To select the hospitals for the study purpose, we decided to study both government and private hospitals in Bhiwani city. Bhiwani city is purposively selected as it has large number of private hospitals where large number of patients visit for their treatment.

For the present study General Hospital is selected in the government hospital category. It has 22 doctors and 80–90 patients (on an average) are treated everyday in different wards. One private hospital is selected on the basis of date of establishment and its large size in terms of indoor facility for patients. Among the list of 46 hospitals/clinic/nursing homes, Chugh Hospital was established in 1979 and it is the oldest among the private hospitals. It also has 10–12 patients per day in indoor ward which is the highest among private hospitals. All the doctors of selected private hospital and government hospital during the specific period, i.e. October 2013 to December 2013 are interviewed. The patients who are staying in the indoor ward for more than three days are selected and interviewed.

The patients who minimally stayed for three days are taken into account. Since the government hospital has a large number of patients, therefore, on the basis of their minimum three days stay criteria, we identified two patients daily and interviewed them and this process was repeated for a period of thirty days, which makes it a total of 60 patients. In the Chug private hospital, we decided to select equal number of patients, i.e. 60 patients. Again from Chugh Hospital also we selected and interviewed the 60 patients on the basis of minimum of three days length of stay in the ward.

We have collected both primary and secondary data. Primary data are collected with the help of interview schedule, focused group interview and case histories from doctors as well as from patients.

People come into direct contact with a health system as patients attended by health care providers. The concept of health is not only an absence of disease, but attainment of positive physical, mental health and social health. Health is not determined only by medical care but also by economic, environmental, social, demographic, hygienic, etc. There have been major improvements in India in terms of infant mortality, maternal mortality, life expectancy; however, the burden of diseases like tuberculosis, HIV infection, malaria, filarial, leprosy is huge. Children are severely affected by under nutrition and diarrhoea.

Health infrastructure in terms of provision of sufficient number of SHC, PHC and CHC and government hospitals are insufficient in number. Availability of doctors, nurses and other paramedical personnel also influence access to care. Drug availability in government hospitals is insufficient and at the same time poor people are not able to pay for the medicine, which in turn affects their health. Further, the infrastructure of health is very poor in rural areas as compared to urban areas as many PHCs and CHCs are without sufficient number of doctors. In urban areas there are 308 beds per 1,00,000 populations as compared to 44 beds per 1,00,000 rural populations. The development of country is measured in terms of health care indicators. The health care development is directly dependent on the programme and policies of the government.

Despite several interventions in health care sector, the health system continues to be inadequate and insufficient to cover the population efficiently. It continues to be disconnected with public health goals, inadequately equipped to address peoples' expectation and fails to provide protection to those unable to access care for want of ability to pay.

The role of public and non-household private sector is considered to be important in reducing the burden of health care expenditure on households. The public expenditure on health is very low. Out of pocket payment in India is approximately 97 per cent of total private expenditure. However, in India, the provision of health under Indian Constitution falls in the state list. That is why there is a great difference in terms of health indicators in different states of the country. To support the health structure of the country, government introduced a three-tier, i.e. primary, secondary and tertiary support structure for addressing the health issues across the country. The aim of health policy is to secure a fundamental change in the health status of its people. In order to do the same the 'Health for All by 2000 AD' was implemented in 1978. The basic task of this movement was to provide a minimum standard of health to its entire people, latest by year 2000. However, the country could not achieve this goal. In 1983, the government had come up with the idea of health policy of 1983 which envisaged the inter-sectoral cooperation like housing, education, rural development, social welfare, water supply, sanitation, etc. Again in 2002, New National Health Policy was designed where preventive and curative initiatives at primary level were encouraged. Emphasis was also laid on rational use of drugs within the allopathic system. Increased access to tried and tested system of traditional medicine was also ensured. In spite of massive development, the rural health care remained ignored. Therefore, in 2005, NRHM was launched for exclusively targeting the rural population for its health care needs.

In Haryana, the health situation of its population is also not very impressive. However, it has a good position in terms of economic development. Number of posts of doctors and other paramedical staff are lying vacant in government hospitals which in turn affect the health care availability to the masses.

There is a mushroomed growth of private health care in urban area and at the same time absence of government health care facilities in rural areas, which is forcing people to go to the urban areas for seeking treatment. Nearly one-third of patients are in the age group of 21–30 years, who are seeking treatment in government and private hospitals. Little less than seventy per cent are married who are seeking treatment in different government and private hospitals. Nearly fifty per cent of the patients in government and private hospitals are from OBC category. Patients from higher income group prefer private hospital for treatment as compared to government hospital. Little more than forty per cent patients are having income between one lakh to three lakh.

Earlier the medical profession was found to be predominantly male dominated; however, in the present society of the overall number of medical professionals, little less than fifty per cent are women. It is so because woman have also started coming into the medical profession like in all other professions. The age-group of the doctors ranges from 25 to 51 years and above. Little more than one-third of the doctors are in the younger age group, i.e. 25–30 years. Examining the rural-urban background of the doctors, we found that nearly eighty per cent of doctors are having an urban background. Urbanization has led to disintegration of joint family system; our study also reveals that nearly seventy per cent of doctors are having a nuclear family structure. All the doctors are married except three doctors, who are thinking of going for higher studies and, therefore, they do not want to get married. More than fifty per cent of doctors are drawn from other backward caste category which includes Jat, Yadav, Khati, Kumhar, Panchal, and Jat Sikh. Only two doctors are from scheduled caste and that too in the government hospital. Since we have taken doctors from government and private hospitals; therefore, we find a mix of doctors from allopathic degree and ayurveda degree. More than one-third of the doctors have their postgraduate degree of MD/MS. Little less than one-third of the doctors have their annual income between five to seven lakh per year. Regarding the experience of the doctors in the hospital, exactly fifty per cent of the doctors have less than five years of experience in that particular health facility.

If people have capacity to pay, then they want to avail the private ward facility within the government hospital. In private hospital, there is a trend that the higher the income group, more the patients opt for a special ward. Thus, it implies that higher income group people are ready to pay for better facilities. Well educated patients go to the private hospital instead of government hospital to take treatment. People who are engaged in different professions avoid seeking treatment in government hospital; however old people, students and unemployed patients are seeking treatment in government hospital. People from joint family prefer to take treatment in government hospital, as they have more members in their household and hence can accompany the patient to government hospital. People do not want to go to private hospital for dental problems as they think that dental treatment is costly. In our study, patients are seeking dental treatment from government hospital. However, for surgery related issues and other diseases they are going to private and government hospitals depending upon their income and level of urgency for the treatment. People have diverse views on concept of health. Nevertheless, a majority of the respondents identified good health with normal functioning of the body, good sound sleep and good appetite. There are other people who also viewed good health in terms of energy level, able to work normally, etc. Some people also give importance to good body build and to the absence of disease and illness in the body. More than eighty per cent of the respondents believe that one should follow a healthy lifestyle to remain healthy and it is individual's responsibility. Forty-five per cent of the patients, who are seeking treatment in government or private hospital, have previously tried Ayurvedic treatment. Nearly forty-four patients have just ignored their illness and therefore, they did not take any treatment before going to the hospital. There are nearly seventy per cent of the patients who did not go anywhere for any sort of check-up unless they suffered from some disease.

Almost sixteen per cent patients in government hospital face problem in admission process, whereas less than two per cent patients face problem in admission in private hospital. It means seeking treatment in government hospital is a cumbersome process. Less than twenty patients who faced problem while getting admission into hospital reported that doctors just ignore the seriousness of their illness. Ten patients experienced that the doctors are more interested in referring them to some other health care facility. Near about ten per cent patients reported that their illness was not of serious nature, therefore, doctors did not take any interest in admitting them. Before coming to the health care facility, people experienced different kind of symptoms which vary from body pain to bleeding. However, majority of them were those who felt extreme pain in their body parts and that is why they had come to the hospital. Some of them felt loss of appetite, weakness in body, urine disorder, etc.

Sixty-three per cent of the patients do not follow the treatment prescribed by the doctors. Little less than thirty per cent said that in case they go to the doctor to consult him, and they do not find him, they leave the treatment midway. In all, less than twenty patients pressurized the doctor for immediate relief, whereas nearly forty-five per cent patients in government hospital do not say anything regarding the treatment process. Nearly eighty per cent patients feel that they are not competent and only doctor is specialized in his profession. More than one-third per cent replied that they do not want to interfere in the process of treatment prescribed by the doctor. More than one-fifth of the respondents feel that the treatment process of some diseases is long and therefore, it will take its own time.

Almost forty-five per cent of the patients are more worried about the life of their loved ones than the money involved and nearly quarter per cent of the patients replied that because they do not have any economic problem, therefore, they are not worried about the cost of treatment. Nearly eleven per cent reported that they are not worried about the cost of treatment as they are getting free treatment for being from below poverty line families, whereas nearly six per cent reported that they are under the reimbursement scheme, therefore they are not worried about the cost of treatment. One-third of the patients take it otherwise that disease and illness are also a part of life and therefore, during the process of life one has to spend on their treatment also.

The illiterate persons as they cannot read and write, therefore, they do not bother about reading the expiry date of medicines. Further, they do not ask any other person who is literate to take note of the expiry date of medicines. There are only one quarter of the respondents who note down the date of expiry of medicines before taking it. It shows that the awareness of reading of the expiry date increases with the level of education. Nearly, three-fourths of the patients who replied that they do not bother to read the expiry date of medicines mentioned certain reasons for not taking care of expiry of medicines. Sixty-five per cent of the patients mentioned that they are not aware of expiry of medicines.

One-third of the patients do not have any knowledge of their health rights. The knowledge of health rights increases with the level of education. The patients who understand health rights expressed their interpretation of health rights as right to live with dignity, government's responsibility to provide health services, free health services, very well diagnosed form of treatment and getting treatment in the emergency/casualty in government hospital. More than ninety per cent patients in government and private hospitals think that patients' health right is to receive treatment. Less than twenty per cent patients replied that every patient has a right of confidentiality of his/her treatment, which means doctor is not supposed to disclose his disease to others. Little more than fifty per cent replied that in case of an emergency, treatment should be given immediately without asking for any fee or any other questions whether in government or in private health facility. Another significant number of patients view health rights in terms of adequate health care. However, the crucial elements of right to health care is not given much importance by patients as only twenty per cent replied that they have a right to ask about the process of treatment, and another twenty patients reported that they have the right to informed consent.

Ninety-seven per cent of the patients have gathered information of health rights from newspapers and television. Another sixty-five per cent of the patients in government and private hospitals collect information about health rights from the hospitals only where they are admitted. Nearly one-third of the patients in government hospitals have taken the help of neighbours for information on health rights. Little more than fifteen per cent of the patients of private hospital gathered information from the posters displayed at various public places. Little more than fifty per cent of the patients believed that it is necessary to disseminate information about health rights in the society, particularly through text books in school and colleges. Only four patients replied that there is no need of dissemination of information of health rights. However, fifty patients replied that they do not know how to disseminate information of health rights. Nearly ninety per cent patients replied that it is the duty of the patient to give that fee to the doctor which is agreed upon or which is written on the board. Sixty-five per cent patients feel that their responsibility lies in giving respect to the doctors.

More than sixty-seven per cent of the patients have no knowledge about consent of treatment. These patients replied that they do not understand the complexity of treatment and only the doctor is competent enough to take decisions for their treatment. Satisfaction from treatment not only helps in the healing process but also provides good interaction and relationship between doctors and patients. Sixty-seven per cent patients reported that they are satisfied with the treatment which they are receiving from the hospital. There is some difference in the degree of satisfaction in government and private hospitals. More number of patients in private hospital are satisfied with the treatment as compared to government hospital. Nearly, seventy per cent of patients are satisfied with doctor's behaviour.

However, little more than twenty-five per cent are not satisfied with doctors' behaviour. The patients who are not satisfied with doctors' behaviour are more from government hospital. Further, the dissatisfaction from the behaviour of doctors is reported in terms of their rude behaviour, discrimination in treatment and doctors not sharing the line of treatment. The level of satisfaction from proper care is high in private hospital as compared to government hospital. Overall dissatisfaction with the facility of health care in government and private hospital is reported by the patients in terms of their multiple responses. The important cause of dissatisfaction comes from the poor hygiene in hospital and dirty bedsheets. Most of the diagnostic tests are delayed or machines are not in order and sometimes they are faulty also. That is why patients have doubt on the diagnostic tests done by the hospital staff. Some of them also reported about the doctor's biasness in treatment. The patients are not treated with dignity and respect.

We asked our respondents to give their views about the equality of health rights. Nearly seventy-four per cent replied that there is a discrepancy in realization of health rights. However, nearly twenty-seven per cent opined that there are equal health rights for all irrespective of their caste, class, age, gender and educational level. The patients who opined that there are no equal rights, among them nearly ninety-two per cent feel that health rights are only meant for rich people and another sixty-seven per cent opined that health rights are exercised by people from higher connection.

Our study confirms that because of the complexity in understanding of medical negligence, majority of the respondents reported that they do not understand the medical negligence committed by doctors. However, little more than thirty per cent understand the medical negligence. Urban patients are more aware of medical negligence as compared to patients who come from rural area.

Is it necessary to share the information regarding the cost of treatment, benefits of treatment, risk in particular treatment process, etc.? These are some of the issues which are important from health rights perspective. In normal circumstances, it is expected that a doctor should share the information regarding the cost of treatment, risk involved in the particular treatment and consequences of the treatment. However, in our study nearly fifty-five per cent patients are not ready to accept that they should have information regarding the treatment process and risks involved. Little more than forty-five per cent do feel that they should have the complete information regarding the cost of treatment, consequences of treatment and risks involved in particular treatment.

Patients' cognition and understanding of health is also reflected in their suggestions for improving the health rights' understanding and their implementation. Nearly eighty per cent replied that there should be display of patients' rights at every gate of the hospital so that people can read them. Another eighty-two patients opined that every treatment card, whether OPD card or Indoor card, should have information about health rights. Nearly, fifty per cent of the patients feel that media can play a significant role in disseminating information about the health rights. Nearly, forty per cent of the patients reported that there should be inclusion of chapter on health rights in the text books at school level and at college level.

There are different levels of malpractices being practised in providing health care to the patients. It varies at the level of doctors, pharmacist, diagnostic centres, etc. When we asked our patients regarding the source of their prescribed medicines, nearly one-quarter of patients replied that they buy these medicines from outside the hospital which although they are supposed to get it from the hospital. However, nearly fifteen per cent from private hospital get medicine from inside the hospital. Nearly, forty-seven per cent of the patients accepted that they paid money on receipt of bill for their treatment process; however little more than fifty-three per cent denied that they ever received any receipt of the money paid for the treatment in the hospital.

Like patients, doctors have their own concept of health which is based on their knowledge which they acquire during their study period and also during their practise of medical profession. We have tried to collect the views of the doctors regarding their concept of health. Maximum number of doctors, i.e. eighty-seven per cent find good health in terms of freedom from disease. A good number of doctors, i.e. seventy-eight per cent state that a good health is viewed in terms of good appetite. Another seventy-three per cent view good health in terms of good posture.

Majority of the doctors, i.e. eighty-two per cent mention that one should not ignore illness and if one falls sick one should immediately report to the doctors. Another sixteen doctors said that regular check-ups are must to remain healthy. Another fifteen doctors feel that eating of balanced diet is must to remain healthy.

Seventy-three per cent of the doctors are motivated by service to mankind and the respect they get in the society. However, fifty-five per cent of doctors confess that medical profession gives them chance to earn more money as compared to other professions. Nearly forty-six per cent of the doctors are motivated by professional satisfaction in treating the patients. It is interesting to note that nearly sixty per cent of the doctors feel that good relationship between doctor and patient helps in the treatment process.

Further, regarding the content of the relationship between doctors and patients, nearly eighty-five per cent of the doctors mention that while interacting with the patient they want to clear the doubts of patients in terms of the disease and the process of treatment. Ultimately the clarity of doubts helps in the treatment process. Nearly seventy per cent doctors view that social interaction with the patient is their social responsibility which helps the healing process. Five of them feel that by having social interaction with the patient, their mental tension is diverted and they are also motivated to act according to professional ethics. Nearly, sixty per cent of the doctors maintain that they have normal behaviour with their patients, whereas fifty per cent of the doctor said that they are cooperative with their patients. Nearly, twenty-three per cent of the doctors are friendly with their patients and another fourteen per cent are emotive with their patients.

Almost, sixty-eight per cent of the doctors mentioned that they know the name of the oath taken by them, whereas nearly thirty per cent do not remember the name of the oath taken by them. These shows that almost one-third of the doctors do not bother to remember the name of the oath. Further, when we asked the doctors to tell about the contents of the oath, seventy per cent of them replied in bits and pieces.

There are five major elements of ethics in the medical profession. They are respect of autonomy of medical professionals, beneficence and non-malfeasance, justice to all patients, informed consent and truthfulness and confidentiality in the medical profession. Nearly seventy-three per cent of the doctors mentioned that autonomy of the doctor is very important in the medical profession. Another sixty-nine per cent of the doctors give priority to informed consent in their profession. Fifty-five per cent doctors maintain that medical profession is basically a profession of beneficence and non-malfeasance. To provide justice to all, irrespective of their strata is another element of ethics in the medical profession.

Professional ethics of a doctor suggest that a doctor is supposed to treat the patient irrespective of his caste, class, ethnic group, gender and other biasness. Forty-one per cent doctors straight away replied that they can refuse treatment, whereas majority of the doctors, i.e. fifty-nine per cent still maintain that they cannot refuse treatment to any patient. The doctors, who refuse to treat the patient, have shared their reasons for it. Nearly, eighty-nine per cent of the doctors say that there is no legal binding on them to treat a patient after their duty hours. Furthermore, seventy per cent of the doctors share that they treat a patient only when they think that it is an emergency; sometimes they have had some bad experience in the past of treating patients after their duty hours. They also refuse to treat patients when there are no facilities available to treat them. Sometimes, doctors also refuse to treat the patient if they are already occupied with the treatment process of some other patient or if they themselves are not well. Some doctors also refuse to treat patients in odd hours.

Fifty per cent of the doctors mentioned diplomatically that it depends upon the situation of the person. However, nearly forty-six per cent of the doctors replied that they will immediately provide first aid to the patient irrespective of any situation. Thirty-six per cent of the doctors mentioned that they will immediately inform their relatives.

We asked doctors very pertinent questions about what constitutes medical ethics. The responses collected from the doctors are varied. Sixty-eight per cent of the doctors maintain that they respect the confidentiality of the patient in terms of the disease as well as about treatment. Nearly sixty-four per cent of the doctors view medical ethics in terms of the health and life of a patient; it is the prime concern of the doctors. Exactly fifty per cent of the doctors feel that it is unfair to use medical knowledge contrary to the laws of humanity. Nearly seventy-five per cent feel that doctors should use their medical power and knowledge for the benefit of the patient. Majority of the doctors, i.e. eighty-two per cent maintain that medical profession is the profession of conscience and dignity.

Out of twenty-two doctors, almost one-third of the doctors admit that there are cases of medical negligence in the medical facilities. However, approximately seventy per cent of the doctors have completely denied that there are any cases of medical negligence in the hospital. Elaborating on the forms of medical negligence, eighty-seven per cent mentioned that taking out of patients' organs without his/her consent is the most severe form of medical negligence. Nearly, seventy-three per cent report that delay in the treatment of the patient is also a form of medical negligence. Nearly seventy per cent feel that wrong treatment is also a type of medical negligence. Overdose of medicine is another form of medical negligence which has been mentioned by sixty-four per cent.

Of the doctors who reported that there are cases of medical negligence in the medical facility, sixty per cent of the doctors opined that many times new medicines are given to the patient on trial basis. This may be due to kick backs from the pharmaceutical companies or may be from the medical representatives of the company who are visiting the doctors for the promotion of their medicines. Another seventy-four per cent of the doctors feel that there is rampant use of medical devices like stent, etc. which are in reality not needed for treatment. Thus, medical negligence is viewed in terms of drug administration to the patients and also unnecessary use of medical devices which are not needed for treating the patients.

Doctors are keen to reply about the medical information they share with their patients. The information which they share with their patients ranges from type of medicine to the side effects of the medicine and procedure of taking it. Maximum numbers of doctors, i.e. eighty-seven per cent, always tell their patients about the side effects of the medicine, whereas sixty-nine per cent of the doctors tell their patients about the full course of the antibiotics. They tell their patients that if you do not take the full course of treatment, your disease might recur shortly. Fourteen doctors told that they never forget to tell their patients about not stopping medicine even when they have recovered. Doctors think that generally patients stop taking prescribed medicine as soon as they feel that they have recovered. Sixty per cent of the doctors tell their patients about the substitutes of the medicines also because sometimes a particular brand of medicine is not available. Telling substitutes of medicines help patients in getting another one if the original is not available.

We learned from our doctors about informed consent and the type of treatment. Eighty-seven per cent of the doctors replied that in case of a surgical treatment informed consent is a must, seventy-three per cent replied in favour of organ transplant and fifty five per cent of the doctors have replied that even in case of a normal treatment informed consent is necessary.

Nearly, fifty-five per cent doctors straight away replied that informed consent is a must even in case of an urgent medical care. However, forty-six per cent patients feel that there is no need to ask the patient for the medical care as treatment is more important than consent.

Regarding the obstacles in taking the consent from the patient, doctors' responses are received in multiple forms. Eighty-four per cent of the doctors feel that it is very difficult to explain the technicality of the treatment to the patients as majority of the patients are either illiterate or they do not have any knowledge of treatment. Similarly, seventy-five per cent of the doctors' opinion is that it is very difficult for them to explain the line of treatment as the language becomes the barrier. Nearly, sixty per cent of the doctors mention that non-availability of relatives/guardian at the time of treatment, patient's inability to talk to the doctor and absence of other methods to inform the patient for the treatment are major obstacles in taking their consent.

Regarding the format of the consent for the treatment, seventy-eight per cent of the doctors said that the consent must be related only to that particular treatment of the diseases which a person is going for. Another, sixty-nine per cent opine that whatever consent they give, it should be communicated to the doctor. There should be no pressure on the patient for giving consent for the treatment. This opinion shared by nearly twenty-eight per cent of doctors. Fifty-five per cent of the doctors strongly believe that consent must not be obtained through fraudulent means or misrepresentation of facts.

Maintaining confidentiality of the patient is another attribute of the medical ethics of doctors. Exactly fifty per cent of the doctors mentioned that they keep their patients' information as confidential, whereas twenty-three per cent of the doctors maintain that it depends upon the situation. Twenty-eight per cent maintain that they do not bother to keep confidentiality of the disease and treatment process of their patients.

Majority of doctors, i.e. seventy-three per cent, mentioned that giving guide lines for the prevention of disease is the best method for better health. Similarly, another sixty-four per cent of the doctors feel that regular medical check-ups and following a healthy lifestyle can make a person healthy. Minimum charges for consulting doctors, cracking down on health care fraud, providing free preventing care and proper rendering of health care are also crucial aspects.

Practice and understanding of health rights can only be understood when we comprehend the views of users of health care as well as from the providers of health care. In our study, maximum number of doctors, i.e. eighty-seven per cent feel that free choice of health services is the most important aspect of health right. However, eighty-two per cent of the doctors feel that the patient's right is to get equal treatment irrespective of his caste, class, ethnic group, economic background and occupational background. Receiving adequate health care is the right of the patients has been mentioned by nearly seventy per cent of the doctors. There are many urgent situations where patient needs immediate care without delay. This has been viewed by sixty-four per cent of the doctors. A large number of doctors also feel that a patient should be treated with dignity and in a welfare state it is the duty of the government to provide health care to its citizens. Some of the doctors view the rights of the patient in terms of getting receipts of medicine, diagnostic tests and fee of doctors.

Nearly fifty-five per cent of the doctors completely favour organ donation. According to them, it can save the life of a person. However, thirty-two per cent of the doctors are quite opposed to the idea of organ donation as they say that it is unethical to take out the organ of one person and transplant it in another person. Furthermore, according to them it will also increase unethical practices in the medical profession. Fourteen per cent of the doctors maintain that donation of organs can be useful in some cases. Donation and transplantation of organs will depend upon the nature and situation of the patient and donor.

A hospital is part of a sophisticated health service. It is connected in thought to a wide network of people and actions that in one way or the other is concerned with maintaining and improving his health for the rest of his life as for the rest of the population. Doctors, policy makers, and nowadays financers for big corporate hospitals and private hospitals together form a health system. Health systems have played a part in the dramatic rise in life expectancy, diagnosis of diseases, treatment of a number of diseases, decreasing percentage of mortality with diseases are some of the manifestations in the 21st century. Medical science has contributed enormously to better health and influenced the lives and well-being of billions of men, women and children around the world. Their role has become increasingly important. With the increasing level of education, knowledge and awareness of people about their health responsibilities, their health behaviour, their process of seeking treatment and of course awareness about health right has also contributed in the wellness of human society.

Where then do the poor go when they do not receive medicines? They have two options – they can wait and suffer or they go to the private sector. Actually, this is not really a choice. It is well-known that a large number of patients seek care in the private sector only due to the overburdened and patient-unfriendly nature of the public sector. So, those who seek care in the public sector either cannot afford to go to the private sector or have already been exploited by it. This raises the critical question of the government's role as the primary provider of drugs and services to the poorest. This extensive power seems to come with little accountability. The issue also has ethical implications: how can the states put lives of patients in danger by not making essential drugs available? Patients suffering from certain diseases also suffer from extensive physical, psychological, social and economic consequences of these diseases. These diseases affect income, raise expenses and often push families into debt. By not providing appropriate and timely treatment, the government is further acerbating their suffering and also limiting their ability to build constructive lives.

The study has broadly analysed health care from two points of view: doctors and patients. There are some general conclusions, which have come up in the study. It is found that there is a difference in government and private hospitals. People are not able to get the best treatment in government hospitals because of unavailability of doctors, rude behaviour and lack of infrastructural facilities. Social position of the individuals, for instance, the kinds of service available for a person depend on the resources at the personal level as well as societal level which pre-exists the personal. Secondly, it can be argued that communication regarding the illness/disease is almost nil. Patients are hardly communicated for their pattern of treatment, unless and until one shows anxiety to know about it. Informed choice for the treatment is conspicuously absent, as patients are hardly informed and in turn patients also think that it is the doctor who is the most competent person to look for treatment. Treatment process cannot be viewed without the patient as the primary concern. Patient should be brought into the centre. The serious issues of treatment should not bypass the patient but it should be a matter of available choices.

Limitation of this Study

We now turn to some limitations of this study which is exploratory and descriptive in nature. The study could have been more intensive and qualitative in nature but due to certain constraints we could not do that. The research sets out the issues which may be purled in details in future regarding the episodic cases of medical negligence, confidentiality, informed choice, etc. The study has not been able to examine the role and activities of pharmaceutical stores and diagnostic centres.

Despite these limitations this piece of research is intended to contribute to the understanding of health rights of patients and ethics of doctors in private and government health care facilities. In this respect, this study should be of interest to sociology and anthropology of medicine, apart from public and private health. It is also a study of the basic rights of human beings, i.e. health of the people.

Appendix

The Hippocratic Oath

It is not certain that the Hippocratic Oath was written by Hippocrates but it was probably written during his lifetime. The earliest surviving reference to this Oath date from the 1st century AD. These suggest that the Oath was seen as an ideal rather than a norm and it was not until the 4th century that it was an obligatory recruitment for the doctor to take the Oath before practising. Perhaps the most enduring tradition in the history of medicine is the Hippocratic Oath. Named after the famous Greek physician Hippocrates, this oath was written as a guideline for the medical ethics of doctors. Although the exact words have changed over time, the general content is the same. An oath to respect those who have imparted their knowledge up on the science of medicine and respect to the patients as well as the promise to treat them to the best of the physician's ability.

I swear by Apollo Physician and Asclepius and Panacea and all the gods and goddesses, making them my witnesses, that I will fulfil according to my ability and judgement this oath and this covenant:

To hold him who has taught me this art as equal to my parents and to live my life in partnership with him and if he is in need of money to give him a share of mine and to regard his offspring as equal to my brothers in male lineage and to teach them this art- if they desire it- without fee and covenant, to give share of precepts and oral instruction and all the other learning to my sons and to the sons of him who has instructed me and to pupils who have signed the covenant have taken oath according to the medical law but no one else.

I will apply dietetic measures for the benefit of the sick according to my ability and judgement; I will keep them from harm and injustice.

I will neither give a deadly drug to anybody if asked for it. Nor will I make a suggestion to this effect. Similarly, I will not give to a woman abortive remedy. In purity and holiness, I will guard my life and my art.

I will not use the knife not even on sufferers from stone, but will withdraw in favour of such as re-engaged in this work.

Whatever houses I may visit, I will come for the benefit of the sick, remaining free of all intentional injustice, of all mischief and in particular of sexual relations with both female and male persons, be they free or slaves.

What I may see or hear in the course of the treatment or even outside of the treatment in regard to the life of men, which on no account one must spread, I will keep to myself holding such things shameful to be spoken about.

If I fulfil this oath and do not violate it, may it be granted to me to enjoy life and art being honoured with fame among all time to come, if I transgress it and swear falsely, may the opposite of all this be my lot. (Source: Ethical codes and declarations to the health professionals, Amnesty International, 2001).

References

Abel-Smith, B. (1976), *Value for Money in Health Services*, London: Heinemann.

Abrams, M. (1968), 'Blueprint for Consumer Satisfaction', in J. McKenzie (ed.), *Consumer and the Health Services*, London: Office of Health Economics.

Advani, Mohan (1980), *Doctor-Patient Relationship in Indian Hospitals*, Jaipur: Sanghi Prakashan.

Anitha, V. (2011), 'Cost of Treatment: A Study Based on Medical Pluralism', in K. Gangadharan (ed.), *Health and Development: The Millennium Perspectives*, Jaipur: Rawat Publications.

Ansari, S.H. (2005), 'Spatial Organization of Health Care Facilities in Haryana', *National Geographical Journal of India*, 51(3–4): 51–62.

Ashraf, A. and Rodrigues, M. (2002), *Private Health Sector in India*, Compiled Monograph, Chapat, Mumbai.

Atkinson, P. (1995), *Medical Talk and Medical Work: The Liturgy of the Clinic*, London: Sage Publications.

Babson, J.H. (1973), 'Disease Costing, Studies in Social Administration', in M.F. Drummond (ed.), *Principles to Economic Appraisal in Health Care*, Oxford: Oxford University Press.

Bajpai, Nirupam (2010), *Improving Access and Efficiency in Public Health Services*, New Delhi: Sage Publications.

Balaraman, C.S. (1990), 'Emergency Services in Hospitals', in S.L. Goel (ed.), *Hospital Administration and Management*, New Delhi: Deep and Deep Publications.

Balint, M. (1971), *The Doctor, His Patient and the Illness*, London: Pitman Medical.

Banerjee, A., Deaton, A. and Duflo, E. (2004), 'Wealth, Health, and Health Services in Rural Rajasthan', *American Economic Review*, 94(2): 326–30.

Banerji, D. (1982), *Poverty, Class and Health Culture in India*, New Delhi: Prachi.

Barber, Bernard et al. (1973), *Research on Human Subjects*, New York: Russell Sage.

Barry, V. (1982), *Moral Aspects of Health Care*, Belmont, CA: Wordsworth.

Baru, R.V. (1998), *Private Health Care in India: Social Characteristics and Trends*, New Delhi: Sage Publications.

Beauchamp, Tom L. and Childress, James E. (1983), *Principles of Biomedical Ethics*, New York: Oxford University Press.

——. (2001), *Principles of Biomedical Ethics*, USA: Oxford University Press.

Bennett, S. et al. (1994), 'Canon and Stick: State Mechanisms to Influence Private Provider Behaviour', *Health Policy and Planning*, 9(1): 1–13.

Bensely, R.J. (1991), 'Defining Spiritual Health: A Review of the Literature', *Journal of Health Education*, 22(5): 287–90.

Berger, J. (1967), *A Fortunate Man*, Harmondsworth: Penguin.

Berger, J. and Mohr, J. (1967), *A Fortunate Man: The Story of a Country Doctor*, London: The Penguin Press, pp. 50–56.

Bhat, R. (1993), 'The Private/Public Mix in Health Care in India', *Health Policy and Planning*, 8(1): 43–56.

Bhatnagar, S., Dosajh, V. and Kapoor, S.D. (1988), 'Utilization of Health Care Facilities in Urban Slums of Delhi', *Health Population Perspective and Issues*, 11(4): 162–70.

Bhattacharya, S.K. and Dipika Sur (2007), 'Ethical Guidelines for Biomedical Research on Human Participants', *Indian Journal of Medical Research*, 126(6), 587–589.

Bhore, Joseph (1946), *Report of the Health Survey and Development Committee*, Volume I to IV, Government of India, Delhi.

Bloom, S.W. (1963), *The Doctor and His Patient*, New York: Russell Sage Foundation.

British Medical Association (1986), *The Handbook of Medical Ethics*, London: BMA.

Brooks, R.G. (1969), 'Cost-Benefit Analysis of Patients Treated at a Rheumatism Centre', *Annuals of Rheumatic Disease*, 28: 665–61.

Burch, Sarah (2001), 'Cultural Studies', in Jennie Naidoo and Jane Wills (eds), *Health Studies: An Introduction*, New York: Palgrave.

Capron, Alexander et al. (1979), *Genetic Counseling: Facts, Values, and Norms*, New York: Alan R. Liss.

Cartwright, A. (1967), *Patients and their Doctors*, London: Routledge and Kegan Paul.

Cemper, G.E. (1984), *Determinants of Health Levels in Developing Countries*, England: Research Studies Press Ltd.

CESCR (Committee on Economic, Social and Cultural Rights) (2000), *General Comment No. 14, 'Right to the Highest Attainable Standard of Health'*, 11 August 2000, UN Doc. E/C.12/2000/4.

Chakraborty, Achin and Mukherjee, Subrata (2003), 'Health Care in West Bengal: What is Happening?', *Economic and Political Weekly*, 38(48): 5021–23.

Chapman, Audrey (1993), *Exploring a Human Rights Approach to Healthcare Reform*, Washington, DC: American Association for the Advancement of Science.

Chapman, Carleton B. (1984), *Physicians, Law and Ethics*, New York: New York University Press.

Chattopadhyaya, D. (1977), *Science and Society in Ancient India*, Kolkata: Research India Publications.

Chaudhury, N. et al. (2003), 'Teacher and Healthcare Providers Absenteeism: A Multicounty Study', Mimeo, Development Research Group, The World Bank.

——. (2006), 'Missing in Action: Teacher and Health Worker Absence in Developing Countries', *Journal of Economic Perspectives*, 20(1): 91–116.

Chauhan, L.S. (2011), 'Public Health in India: Issues and Challenges', *Indian Journal of Public Health*, 55(2): 88–91.

Coleman, J.C. (1974), *Contemporary Psychology and Effective Behaviour*, Glenview, IL: Scott, Foresman.

Cook, H. (2004), 'Historical Keywords: Health', *Lancet*, 364: 1481.

Cooper, B.S. and Rice, D.P. (1976), 'The Economic Cost of Illness Revisited', *Social Security Bulletin*, US Department of Health, Education and Welfare, February.

Crane, Diana (1975), *The Sanctity of Social Life: Physicians' Treatment of Critically Ill Patients*, New York: Russell Sage.

Croog, Sydney H. and Levine, Sol (1982), *Life After a Heart Attack*, New York: Human Sciences Press.

——. (2002), *India's Development and Participation*, New Delhi: Oxford University Press.

Daniels, Norman and Sabin, J.E. (2002), 'Strengthening the Consumer Voice in Managed Care: IV', *The Philadelphia Consumer Satisfaction Programme, Psychiatric Series*, 53(4): 405–11.

Das, J. and Hammer, J. (2007), 'Money for Nothing: The Dire Straits of Medical Practice in Delhi, India', *Journal of Development Economics*, 83(1): 1–36.

Deaton, A. and Dreze, J. (2009), 'Food and Nutrition in India: Facts and Interpretations', *Economic and Political Weekly*, 44(7): 42–45.

Desai, Mihir and Chand, Dipti (2007), 'Right to Emergency Health Care', in Mihir Desai and Kamayani Bali Mahabal (eds), *Health Care Case Law in India: A Reader*, Mumbai: CEHAT.

Desai, Prakash N. (1988), 'Medical Ethics in India', *The Journal of Medicine and Philosophy*, 13(3): 231–55.

DGHS (2014), *Haryana Health Services at a Glance 2012–2013*, Panchkula, Haryana.

Djukanovic, V. and Mach, E.P. (eds) (1975), *Alternative Approaches to Meeting Basic Health Needs in Developing Countries*, Geneva: World Health Organisation.

Dreze, Jean and Sen, Amartya (1989), *Hunger and Public Action*, Oxford: Clarendon Press.

Duggal, R. (1999), 'Healthcare Utilisation in India', *Health Millions*, 2(1): 10–12.

Duggal, Ravi and Gangolli, Leena (2005), *Review of Healthcare in India*, Mumbai: CEHAT.

Elliot, P. (1972), *The Sociology of the Profession*, London: Macmillan, p. 83.

Emanuel, E.J. and Dubler, N.N. (1995), 'Preserving the Physician-Patient Relationship in the Era of Managed Care', *JAMA*, 273(4): 323–29.

Evans, Timothy (2001), *Challenging Inequalities in Health: From Ethics to Action*, New York: Oxford University Press.

Faden, R. and Faden, A. (1978), 'The Ethics of Health Education as Public Health Policy', *Health Education Monographs*, 6(2): 180–97.

Feldstein, M. (1970), 'The Rising Prices of Physicians Services', *Review of Economics and Statistics*, 52(2): 121–33.

Fidler, David P. (1999), *International Law and Infectious Diseases*, Oxford: Clarendon.

FMRAI (Federation of Medical Representative Association of India) (2001), 'Note on Amendment to the Drug Price Control Order, 1995', presented at the National Drug Convention, New Delhi, 14 June.

Foucault, M. (1990), *La Vida de los Hombres Infamies*, Madrid: Ediciones la Piqueta.

Fox, Renee C. (1974), 'Ethical and Existential Developments in Contemporary American Medicine: Their Implications for Culture and Society', *Milbank Memorial Fund Quarterly*, 52: 445–83.

Freidson, E. (1961), *Patients' Views of Medical Practice*, New York: Russell Sage Foundation, p. 167.

Fuchs, Victor R. (1981), 'Economics, Health and Post-Industrial Society', in John B. McKinlay (ed.), *Economics and Health Care*, Cambridge: MIT Press, pp. 12–27.

Gangadharan, K. and Chandran, K.P. Vipin (2008), 'Nutritional Deprivation among Indian Children: Distributional Profile and Implications', *Journal of the Institute for Research in Social Sciences and Humanities*, 3(1): 85–97.

Ghosh, B.N. (2001), *From Market Failure to Government Failure*, Leeds: Wisdom House.

Gilligan, C. (1982), *In a Different Voice: Psychological Theory and Women's Development*, Cambridge, Massachusetts: Harvard University Press.

Goel, Rajneeesh (2002), *Community Health Care*, New Delhi: Deep and Deep Publications.

Goel, S.L. and Kumar, R. (1990), *Hospital Administration and Management*, New Delhi: Deep and Deep Publications.

Good, B.J. and Good, M.D. (2000), 'Clinical Narratives and the Contemporary Doctor-Patient Relationships', in G. Albrecht, R. Fitzpatrick and S.

Schrimshaw (eds), *Handbook of Social Studies in Health and Medicine*, London: Sage Publications, pp. 243–58.

Goode, William J. and Hatt, P.K. (1981), *Methods in Social Research*, New Delhi: McGraw Hill Books Company.

Gopal, Reema (2004), *Multipurpose Workers in the Context of Primary Healthcare*, Ph.D. Thesis, University of Delhi.

Gottlieb, N., Burdine, J. and McLeroy, K. (eds) (1987), 'Ethical Dilemmas in Health Promotion', *Health Education Quarterly*, 14 (Spring): 1–109.

Government of India (1983), *Statement on National Health Policy 1982*, New Delhi: Ministry of Health and Family Welfare.

——. (2002), National Health Policy, New Delhi: Ministry of Health and Family Welfare.

——. (2005), *National Rural Health Mission*, New Delhi: Indian Public Health Standards for Community Health Centres.

——. (2006), *Approach Paper to the Eleventh Five-Year Plan*, New Delhi: Planning Commission.

Gupta, D. (1988), 'For a Sociology/Anthropology of Illness: Towards a Delineation of its Disciplinary Specificities', *International Sociology*, 3(4): 403–13.

Harron, Frank, Burnside, John and Beauchamp, Tom (1983), *Health and Human Values: A Guide to Making Your Own Decisions*, New Haven: Yale University Press.

Hasan, Khwaja Arif (1979), *Medical Sociology of Rural India*, Ajmer: Sachin Publications.

Haynes, R. (1991), 'Inequalities in Health and Health Service Use: Evidence from the General Household Survey', *Social Science and Medicine*, 33: 361–68.

Hedgecoe, A.M. (2006), 'It's Money that Matters: The Financial Context of Ethical Decision Making in Modern Biomedicine', *Social Health Illness*, 28: 768–84.

Herzlich, C. and Pierret, J. (1987), *Illness and Self in Society*, translated by E. Forster, Baltimore: Johns Hopkins University Press.

Hessler, Kristen and Buchanan, Allen (2002), 'Specifying the Content of the Human Right to Healthcare', in Rosamond Rhodes et al. (eds), *Medicine and Social Justice: Essays on the Distribution of Healthcare*, New York: Oxford University Press, pp. 84–85.

Hiremath, Vijay and Mahabal, Kamayani Bali (2007), 'Reproductive Rights', in Mihir Desai and Kamayani Bali Mahabal (eds), *Health Care Case Law in India: A Reader*, Mumbai: CEHAT.

Hoff, L.A. (1989), *People in Crisis: Understanding and Helping*, Redwood City, CA: Addison-Wesley.

Hughes, E.C. (1958), *Men and their Work*, London: Collier-Macmillan.

ICSSR and ICMR (1981), *Health for All: An Alternative Strategy*, Report of a Study Group, Pune: Indian Institute of Education.

IIPS and Macro International (2008), *National Family Health Survey (NFHS-3), India, 2005–06: Fact Sheets of India and the States*, Mumbai: IIPS.

India's Public Health System (2004), 'How Well Does it Function at the National Level?', *World Bank Policy Research Working Paper*, No. 3447, November.

International Covenant on Economic, Social and Cultural Rights (1966), *United Nations, Treaty Series*, Vol. 933, 19 December, p. 3.

Iyer, A. and Sen, G. (2000), 'Health Sector Changes and Health Equity in the 1990s', in Shobha Raghuram (ed.), *Health and Equity-Effecting Change*, Bangalore (now Bangaluru): HIVOS.

Jesani, Amar (1995), 'Law, Ethics and Medical Council: Evolution of their Relationships', *Medical Ethics*, 3(3), July–September: 9–12.

Kane, Robert L. et al. (1985), 'Hospital's Role in Alleviating the Emotional Stress of Terminal Patients and their Families', *Medical Care*, 23: 189–97.

Khan, Sheeraj Latif Ahmad (1995), 'Right to Health', *Supreme Court Journal*, 2: 29.

Khandekar, S. (2011), 'Health Care Within the Common Man's Reach', *Prayas*, 1: 21.

Kleinman, A. (1978), 'Concepts and a Model for the Comparison of Medical Systems as Cultural Systems', *Social Science and Medicine*, 12: 85–93.

Knowles, John (1977), 'The Responsibility of the Individuals', in J.H. Knowles (ed.), *Doing Better and Feeling Worse*, New York: W.W. Norton, pp. 57–80.

Krishnan, T.N. (1994), 'Access to Health and Burden of Treatment in India: An Inter-State Comparison', *Studies on Human Development in India*, Project of the UNDP, Discussion Paper Series No. 2, CDS, Thiruvanthapuram.

——. (1999), 'Access to Health and the Burden of Treatment in India: An Inter-State Comparison', in M. Rao (ed.), *Disinvesting in Health: The World Bank's Prescriptions for Health*, New Delhi: Sage Publications.

Krishnaswami, P. (2004), 'Morbidity Study: Incidence, Prevalence, Consequences and Associates', *Kerala Research Programme on Local Development*, Discussion Paper No. 63, CDS, Thiruvanthapuram.

Kumar, R. (2008), *Challenges of Healthcare in India*, New Delhi: Deep and Deep Publications.

——. (2011), *Health and Human Development*, New Delhi: Deep and Deep Publications.

Kumar, S. (2003), 'News Roundup: Health Care is Among the Most Corrupt Services in India', *British Medical Journal*, 326: 10.

Kumar, S. Vijaya (1996), 'Rural Elderly: Health Status and Available Health Services', *Research and Development Journal*, 2(3): 16–22.

Lalitha, N. (2007), 'Government Intervention and Prices of Medicine: Lessons from Tamil Nadu', *Working Paper*, No. 175, Gujarat Institute of Development Research, Ahmedabad, July.

Larsen, D.E. and Rootman, I. (1976), 'Physician's Role Performance and Patient Satisfaction', *Social Science and Medicine*, 10: 29–32.

Leary, V.A. (1997), 'Human Rights and the Renewal Agenda', in Z. Bankowski, J.H. Bryant and J. Gallagher (eds), *Ethics, Equity and Health for All*, Geneva: Council for International Organisation of Medical Sciences.

Levine, Sol and Croog, Sydney H. (1985), 'Quality of Life and the Patient's Response to Treatment', *Journal of Cardiovascular Pharmacology*, 7(1): 132–36.

Levine, Sol and Scotch, Norman A. (1970), 'Dying as an Emerging Social Problem', in O.G. Brim, H.E. Freeman, S. Levine and N.A. Scotch (eds), *The Dying Patient*, New York: Russell Sage, pp. 211–22.

Lipkin, M., Putnam, S.M. and Lazare, A. (eds) (1995), *The Medical Interview: Clinical Care, Education, and Research*, New York: Springer.

Madan, T.N. (1972), 'Doctors in a North Indian City: Recruitment, Role Perception and Role Performance', in Satish Saberwal (ed.), *Beyond the Village*, Shimla: Indian Institute of Advanced Study.

——. (1980), *Doctor and Society: Three Asian Case Studies – India, Malaysia and Sri Lanka*, New Delhi: Vikas Publishing House.

Mann, Jonathan et al. (1994), 'Health and Human Rights', *Health and Human Rights*, 1(1): 7–23.

Mathiharan, Karunakaran (2006), 'Supreme Court on Medical Negligence', *Economic and Political Weekly*, XLI(2), 14 January.

Mathur, Indu and Sharma, Sanjay (1995), *Health Hazards, Gender and Society*, Jaipur: Rawat Publications.

McDowell, I. and Newell, C. (1987), 'The Theoretical and Technical Foundations of Health Measurement', in I. McDowell and C. Newell (eds), *Measuring Health: A Guide to Rating Scales and Questionnaires*, New York: Oxford University Press, pp. 10–42.

Mechanic, David (1968), *Medical Sociology: A Selective View*, New York: Free Press.

——. (1979), *Further Issues in Health Care: Social Policy and the Rationing of Medical Services*, New York: Free Press.

Mechanic, David (ed.) (1983), *Handbook of Health, Health Care and the Health Professors*, New York: Free Press.

Mechanic, David and Aiken, I. (1986), *Application of Social Science to Clinical Medicine and Health Policy*, New Brunswick, NJ: Rutgers University Press.

Medical Council of India (2002), *Professional Conduct, Etiquette and Ethics*, Published in Part-3 *Gazette of India*, New Delhi, 6 April.

Merton, R.K. (1957), 'Some Preliminaries to Sociology of Medical Education', in R.K. Merton et al. (eds), *The Student-Physician*, Cambridge: Harvard University Press.

Ministry of Health and Family Welfare (2005), *Report of the National Commission on Macroeconomics and Health*, Government of India, New Delhi.

——. (2011), *Rural Health Statistics Bulletin 2010*, Government of India, New Delhi.

Minocha, Anita (2010), 'Informed Consent in Medical Practice', in B.S. Baviskar and Tulsi Patel (eds), *Understanding Indian Society: Past and Present*, New Delhi: Orient Blackswan.

Mohanty, S.K. and Pathak, P.K. (2009), 'Rich-Poor Gap in Utilization of Reproductive and Child Health Services in India, 1992–2005', *Journal of Biosocial Science*, 41(3): 381–98.

Mooij, J. and Dev, M. (2002), 'Social Sector Priorities: An Analysis of Budgets and Expenditures in India in the 1990s', *Development Policy Review*, 22(1): 97–120.

Morsink, J. (1999), *The Universal Declaration of Human Rights: Origin, Drafting and Intent*, Philadelphia: University of Pennsylvania Press.

Motashaw, Nerges D. (1997), 'Root Causes of Maternal Mortality: Infancy to Motherhood', *Journal of Family Welfare*, 43(2), June.

Nagla, Madhu (1980), *Sociology of Medical Profession: A Study of Doctors at Medical College Hospital*, Rohtak, M.A. Dissertation, M.D. University, Rohtak.

——. (1988), *Medical Sociology: A Study of Professionals and their Clients*, Jaipur: Printwell Publishers.

——. (1993), 'Health Policy and Planning in India', in B.K. Nagla (ed.), *Development and Transformation: Themes and Variations in Indian Society*, Jaipur: Rawat Publications.

——. (1997), *Sociology of Medical Profession*, Jaipur: Rawat Publications.

Nandraj, S. and Duggal, R. (1997), *Physical Standards in the Private Health Sector: A Case Study of Rural Maharashtra*, Mumbai: Centre for Enquiry into Health and Allied Themes.

National Institute of Health and Family Welfare (2010), *Guidelines for Multipurpose Health Worker (Male)*, Government of India, New Delhi.

National Rural Health Mission (2009), *Fact Sheet States and Union Territories*, Mumbai: International Institute for Population Sciences.

Nayak, R.K. (2004), 'Medical Negligence, Patients Safety and the Law', *Regional Health Forum*, 8(2).

Nozick, Robert (1974), *Anarchy, State and Utopia*, New York: Basic Books.

NSSO (2006), 'Morbidity, Health Care and the Condition of the Aged, National Sample Survey', 60th Round, Report No. 507, Ministry of Statistics and Programme Implementation, Government of India, New Delhi, January–June.

Nuffield Provincial Hospitals Trust (1965), *Waiting in Outpatient Departments: Survey of Outpatient Appointment Systems*, Oxford: Oxford University Press.

Nundy, M. (2005), 'The Not-for-Profit Sector in Medical Care in Financing and Delivery of Health Care Services in India', *National Commission on Macroeconomics and Health Background Papers*, Ministry of Health and Family Welfare, Government of India, New Delhi.

Nussbaum, Maratha (1997), 'Capabilities and Human Rights', *Fordham Law Review*, 66, November: 273–300.

Pachauri, Saroj (1994), 'Women's Reproductive Health in India: Research Needs and Priorities', in Joel Gittelsohn et al. (eds), *Listening to Women Talk About their Health: Issues and Evidence from India*, New Delhi: Har-Anand.

Pandit, M.S. and Pandit, Shobha (2009), 'Medical Negligence: Coverage of the Profession, Duties, Ethics, Case Law, and Enlightened Defense – A Legal Perspective', *Indian Journal of Urology*, 25(3), July–September: 372–78.

Park, J.F. and Park, K. (1990), *Textbook on Preventive and Social Medicine*, Jabalpur: Banarsidas, p. 33.

Parsons, T. (1951), *The Social System*, New York: Free Press.

Pelto, Pretti, J. and Pelto, Gretel H. (1978), *Anthropological Research: The Structure of Inquiry*, Cambridge: Cambridge University Press.

Pendleton, D. and Hasler, J. (eds) (1983), *Doctor-Patient Communication*, London: Academic Press.

Perrin, K.M. and McDermott, R.J. (1997), 'The Spiritual Dimension of Health: A Review', *American Journal of Health Studies*, 13(2): 90–99.

Phadke, Anant (1998), *Drug Supply and Use: Towards a Rational Policy in India*, New Delhi: Sage Publications.

——. (2011), 'Planning Healthcare for All', *Economic and Political Weekly*, 46(21), 21–27 May.

Premi, M.K. (2001), 'The Missing Girl Child', *Economic and Political Weekly*, 26, May, 1875–80.

Press, E. (2000), 'Human Rights: The Next Step', *The Nation*, 25 December: 13–18.

Purohit, Brijesh C. and Siddique, Tasleem (1994), 'Utilization of Health Services in India', *Economic and Political Weekly*, 29(17).

Qadeer, I., Sen, K. and Nayar, K.R. (2001), *Public Health and the Poverty of Reforms: The South Asian Predicament*, New Delhi: Sage Publications.

Radley, A. (1994), *Making Sense of an Illness*, London: Sage Publications.

Ram, F. (2011), 'A Discourse on Human Rights Approach to Maternal and Child Health in India', *Demography India*, 40, January–June: 1–15.

Rani, M., Bonu, S. and Harvey, S. (2007), 'Differentials in the Quality of Ante Natal Care in India', *International Journal for Quality in Health*, pp. 1–10.

Rao, P.S. (1981), *Study on Socio-economical and Demographic Correlation of Medical Care Utilization and Health Behaviour*, Research Report, New Delhi: ICSSR.

Rao, S., Nundy, M. and Dua, A.S. (2005), 'Delivery of Health Services in the Private Sector: Financing and Delivery of Health Care Services in India', *National Commission on Macroeconomics and Health Background Papers*, Ministry of Health and Family Welfare, Government of India, New Delhi.

Ray, O. (2004), 'How the Mind Hurts and Heals the Body', *American Psychologist*, 59: 29–40.

Reddy, Ranga (1995), *Health Care Services Management for Underprivileged*, New Delhi: Delta Publishing House, pp. 135–41.

Reichert, E. (2001), 'Placing Human Rights at the Center of the Social Work Profession', *Journal of Intergroup Relations*, 28(1), Spring: 43–50.

Ritzer, G. and Walczack, D. (1988), 'Rationalization and the De-professionalization of Physicians', *Social Forces*, 67(1): 1–22.

Rodwin, M. (1993), *Medicine, Money and Morals: Physicians' Conflicts of Interest*, New York: Oxford University Press.

Rosenstock, I.M. (1974), 'The Health Belief Model and Preventive Behaviour', *Health Education Monograph*, 2: 354–86.

Ruger, Jennifer Prah (2006), 'Rethinking Equal Access; Agency, Quality and Norms', *Global Public Health*, 2(1): 78–96.

——. (2013), 'Toward a Theory of a Right to Health: Capacity and Incompletely Theorized Agreements', *Yale Journal of Law and the Humanities*, 18(2): 274.

Sakthivel, S. (2005), 'Access to Essential Drugs and Medicines: Financing and Delivery of Health Care Services in India', *National Commission on Macroeconomics and Health Background Papers*, Ministry of Health and Family Welfare, Government of India, New Delhi.

Sandel, Michael J. (1982), *Liberalism and the Limits of Justice*, Cambridge: Cambridge University Press.

Saris, J.A. (1995), 'Telling Stories: Life Histories, Illness Narratives and Institutional Landscapes', *Culture, Medicine and Psychiatry*, 19(1): 39–72.

Sarma, E.A.S. (2004), 'Is Rural Economy Breaking Down? Farmers' Suicides in Andhra Pradesh', *Economic and Political Weekly*, 39(28): 3087–89.

Satia, J., Mavalankar, D. and Bhat, R. (1999), 'Progress and Challenges of Health Sector: A Balance Sheet', *Working Paper 99–10–08*, Indian Institute of Management, Ahmedabad, October.

Sen, A.K. (1999), 'Health in Development', *Bulletin of the World Health Organization*, 77: 619–23.

Sen, Amartya (1988), 'Freedom of Choice: Concepts and Content', *European Economic Review*, 32: 269–94.

——. (1993), 'Capability and Well-being', in M. Nussbaum and A. Sen (eds), *The Quality of Life*, Oxford: Clarendon Press, pp. 30–53.

——. (2004), 'Elements of a Theory of Human Rights', *Philosophy and Public Affairs*, 32(4), Fall.

Silberfarb, Peter M., Philibert, Dawn and Levine, Peter M. (1980), 'Psychological Aspects of Neoplastic Disease II: Affective and Cognitive Aspects of Chemotherapy in Cancer Patients', *American Journal of Psychiatry*, 137: 597–601.

Simmons, R. and DiCanio, M. (1979), 'Biology, Technology and Health', in H. Freeman, S. Levine and L. Reeder (eds), *Handbook of Medical Sociology*, Englewood Cliffs, NJ: Prentice-Hall, pp. 150–73.

Smith, G.D., Bartley, M. and Blane, D. (1990), 'The Black Report on Socio-economic Inequalities in Health 10 Years on', *British Medical Journal*, 301: 373–77.

Smith, R., Hiatt, H. and Berwick, D. (1999), 'Shared Ethical Principles for Everybody in Health Care: A Working Draft from the Tavistock Group', *British Medical Journal*, 318, 23 January: 248–51.

Sontag, S. (1989), *AIDS and Its Metaphors*, London: Penguin.

Sriram, T.G. et al. (1991), 'Informed Consent: A Study of Experiences and Opinion of Utilizers of Health Services from India', *Social Science and Medicine*, 32(12): 1389–92.

Stacey, Margaret (1985), 'Medical Ethics and Medical Practice: A Social Science View', *Journal of Medicine Ethics*, 11: 14–18.

Stiglitz, J. (1998), 'The Role of Government in the Contemporary World', in Vito Tanzi and Ke-young Chu (eds), *Income Distribution and High-quality Growth*, Cambridge: MIT Press, pp. 34–50.

Stimson, Gerry and Webb, Barbara (1975), *Going to See the Doctor*, London: Routledge and Kegan Paul.

Sundar, Ramamani (1995), 'Household Survey of Health Care Utilization and Expenditure', *Working Paper*, No. 53, New Delhi: NCAER.

Susser, M., Watson, W. and Hopper, K. (1985), *Sociology in Medicine*, New York: Oxford University Press.

Tassano, Fabian (1995), *The Power of Life or Death: Medical Coercion and the Euthanasia Debate*, Oxford: London.

Tavistock Group (1999), 'A Shared Statement of Ethical Principle for Those Who Shape and Give Health Care', *British Medical Journal*, 318: 249–51.

The Hindu (2011A), 'AIIMS has No Facility to Treat Her, Alka Back in Kanpur', 29 October 2011, New Delhi.

——. (2011B), 'Who Said Doctors Can't be Ethical and Successful?', 17 July 2011, New Delhi.

The Indian Express (2013), 'Health Chief, to Pay Rs 2 Lakh for Medical Negligence', 12 September 2013, Chandigarh.

The Times of India (1990), 'Putting the Patient at the Heart of it', 18 January 1990, New Delhi, p. 9.

——. (1995), 'Medical Negligence under Consumer Protection Act', 25 November 1995, New Delhi.

——. (2003), 'Free Health Services for 60-plus in Haryana', 28 October 2003, Chandigarh.

——. (2004), 'Whose Life is it, Anyway?', 11 September 2004, New Delhi, p. 11.

——. (2006), 'Will National Rural Health Mission Ever Take Off?', 8 January 2006, New Delhi.

——. (2011A), 'Haryana Faces Lack of Health Infrastructure, Doctors', 11 November 2011, Chandigarh.

——. (2011B), 'India Aims to have a Doctor for Every 1,000 People by 2031', 7 March 2011, New Delhi.

——. (2012), 'VIPs are Ok, but What About Common Man?', 15 August 2012, New Delhi.

——. (2013A), '436 Killed in Clinical Trials Last Year', 24 February 2013, New Delhi.

——. (2013B), 'Unnecessary Stent Usage Worries Doctors Across India', 30 January 2013, New Delhi.

——. (2013C), '2,644 Died During Clinical Trial of Drugs in 7 Years', 26 April 2013, New Delhi.

The Tribune (2007), 'Hospital Told to Pay for Failed Surgery', 14 November 2007, Chandigarh.

——. (2013), 'Compensation Procedures for Death, Injury Notified', 4 February 2013, New Delhi.

Turner, B. (1987), *Medical Power and Social Knowledge*, London: Sage Publications.

Umashankar, P.K. and Misra, Girish (eds) (1993), *Urban Health System*, New Delhi: Reliance Publishing House.

UNICEF (2008), *Tracking Progress in Maternal, Newborn and Child Survival: The 2008 Report, V2, Countdown to 2015: Maternal, Newborn and Child Survival*, New York: United Nations Children's Fund.

United Nations (1948), *Universal Declaration of Human Rights*, Adopted 10 December 1948, GA. Res. 217 AIII, United Nations Document, New York: UN.

Venkatratnam, R. (1979), *Medical Sociology in an Indian Setting*, Madras (now Chennai): Macmillan Co. of India Limited.

VHAI (Voluntary Health Association of India) (1993), *Trading of Organs: Need for a Comprehensive Policy*, New Delhi: VHAI.

Viner, Jacob (1953), *Report of the Committee for Economic Development*, S.H. Ruttenberg, American Federation of Labour and Congress, p. 100.

Waitzkin, H. (1979), 'Medicine, Superstructure and Micropolitics', *Social Science and Medicine*, 13A(6): 601–09.

Waitzkin, H. and Stoeckle, J.D. (1972), 'The Communication of Information about Illness', *Advances in Psychosomatic Medicine*, 8: 180–215.

Walters, LeRoy (1975), *Bibliography of Bioethics*, Detroit: Gale Research Company.

Walzer, Michael (1990), 'The Communication Critique of Liberalism', *Political Theory*, 18(1), February: 6–23.

Weiler, Philip G. (1987), 'The Public Health Impact of Alzheimer's Disease', *American Journal of Public Health*, 77: 1157–58.

WHO (1974), 'Constitution of the World Health Organization', *Chronicle of the World Health Organization*, 1: 29–43.

——. (1986), *Ottawa Charter for Health Promotion, 1986*, Geneva: World Health Organization.

——. (1988), *Managing System for Better Health Facilitator Guide*, Geneva: World Health Organization.

——. (1991), *Maternal Mortality: A Global Fact Book, Division of Family Health*, Geneva: World Health Organization.

——. (2000), *World Health Report: Health System Improving Performance*, Geneva: World Health Organization.

——. (2001), *Macro-Economics and Health: Investing in Health for Economic Development*, Report of the Commission on Macro-Economics and Health, Geneva.

——. (2003), *Shaping the Future: World Health Report 2000*, Geneva: World Health Organization.

——. (2005), *Country Profile*, http://whosea.org/cntryhealth/india/index.htm

——. (2009), *Country Health Profile India*, Regional Office for South-East Asia (SEARO).

Wig, K.L. (1985), ' Medical and Ethical Issues of Population: Reflection of a Physician', delivered a keynote address in the Plenary Session on 23 February 1985 in *World Congress of Law and Medicine*, New Delhi.

Wikler, Daniel (1978), 'Persuasion and Coercion for Health', *Health and Society*, 56(3): 303–38.

World Bank (2001), *India's Future Health Systems: Issues and Options*, Draft Report, New Delhi: World Bank.

World Development Report (1993), *Investing in Health*, New Delhi: Oxford University Press, pp. 108–110.

World Health Report (2000), *Health Systems: Improving Performance*, Geneva: World Health Organization.

World Health Report (2003), *Shaping the Future*, Geneva: World Health Organization.

Yesudian, C.A.K. (1981), 'Differential Utilization of Health Services in Metropolitan City', *Indian Journal of Social Work*, 12(4).

Zarit, Steven H. et al. (1985), *The Hidden Victims of Alzheimer's Disease: Families under Stress*, New York: New York University Press.

Index